Systems Neuroscience and Rehabilitation

Kenji Kansaku · Leonardo G. Cohen
Editors

Systems Neuroscience and Rehabilitation

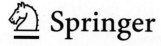 Springer

Editors
Kenji Kansaku
Chief
Systems Neuroscience Section
Department of Rehabilitation
for Brain Functions
Research Institute of National
Rehabilitation Center for Persons
with Disabilities (NRCD)
4-1 Namiki, Tokorozawa
Saitama 359-8555, Japan
kansaku-kenji@rehab.go.jp

Leonardo G. Cohen
Chief
Human Cortical Physiology
and Stroke Neurorehabilitation Section
National Institute of Neurological
Disorders and Stroke (NINDS)
National Institutes of Health (NIH)
10 Center Drive, Bethesda
MD 20892-1430, USA
cohenl@ninds.nih.gov

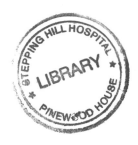

ISBN 978-4-431-53998-8   e-ISBN 978-4-431-54008-3
DOI 10.1007/978-4-431-54008-3
Springer Tokyo Dordrecht Heidelberg London New York

Library of Congress Control Number: 2011930550

Springer is part of Springer Science+Business Media (www.springer.com)

Foreword

It was not so long ago that there was considerable nihilism about the possible treatment of patients with stroke and neurodegenerative conditions. Times have changed. It is now recognized that these patients can, and should, be treated. It is clear that we are able to improve quality of life even if the underlying condition is difficult to cure completely.

Treatment is possible on many different levels. One of the most exciting areas in modern medicine is genetic approaches, but these often seem far in the future. Considerable success has come with manipulation of neurotransmitters, but in order to be successful with this type of therapy there often has to be some derangement in neurotransmitter function to begin with. It is also clear that it is possible to influence the brain at a systems level. One of the most successful types of treatment in this regard is deep brain stimulation. By manipulating different deep nuclei there can be improvement in movement disorders and even psychiatric disorders.

Better understanding of systems neuroscience can lead to other methods of neurorehabilitation. This is the basic premise and theme of the current book. A good example of this concept, and an active area of current rehabilitation research, is the brain–computer interface. By understanding how the brain motor system regulates movement it is possible to capture those signals and relay them to appropriate interfaces to help patients interact with their environment. The brain–computer interface is one of the topics discussed in this book.

Another area of systems neuroscience that is leading to advances in rehabilitation is brain plasticity. By using brain plasticity it is possible to alter brain function. This has been exploited with special types of training and with the relatively new tool of repetitive transcranial magnetic stimulation. Tools like repetitive transcranial magnetic stimulation may even be able to alter the nature of plasticity itself.

The field is moving rapidly and it is difficult to keep up with all the advances. We should all be grateful to Dr. Kenji Kansaku and his colleagues for giving us this useful book, which should be helpful for all health care workers interested in rehabilitation.

Bethesda   Mark Hallett, M.D.
May 2011   Human Motor Control Section
                                                Medical Neurology Branch
                                                National Institute of Neurological
                                                Disorders and Stroke (NINDS)
                                                National Institutes of Health (NIH)

Preface

The brain is an extremely complex system. Disabilities caused by impaired brain function have been tackled mainly from the perspective of rehabilitation, which involves assisting persons with disabilities to recover from or improve dysfunctions, and ultimately aims to improve their well-being. Although much effort has been made to this end, the impaired brain is often difficult to rehabilitate, and part of this difficulty may be caused by our limited knowledge of the mechanisms of the brain system.

Systems neuroscience is a subdiscipline of neuroscience that studies brain functions at the systems level. Recently, advanced techniques have provided new methods for conducting research in this field. For example, imaging techniques such as functional magnetic resonance imaging (fMRI) and magnetoencephalography (MEG) have allowed researchers to investigate spatiotemporal dynamics in the living human brain. Consequently, knowledge in the field is now rapidly growing. In addition, these advanced imaging techniques have started to contribute to the support of impaired brain functions by providing new prosthetics, such as brain–machine and brain–computer interfaces.

The accumulating knowledge in systems neuroscience and related fields might be used for more practical applications in rehabilitation. To discuss this possibility, we launched the Conference on Systems Neuroscience and Rehabilitation in March 2010. The first conference, SNR2010, was held at the National Rehabilitation Center for Persons with Disabilities (NRCD) in Tokorozawa, Japan, and a wide range of researchers from systems neuroscience, neurology, psychology, engineering, and other disciplines exchanged ideas at this forum.

At the conference, keynote and special lectures were given by Dr. Leonardo Cohen of the National Institute of Neurological Disorders and Stroke, Dr. Yves Rossetti of the Université Claude Bernard, and Dr. Shigeru Kitazawa of Juntendo University. After the keynote lecture about brain–computer interfaces and neurorehabilitation by Dr. Cohen, the special lecturers and speakers gave presentations in three sessions: brain–machine or brain–computer interfaces (Dr. Yasuharu Koike of Tokyo Institute of Technology and I), neurorehabilitation (Dr. Toru Ogata of NRCD and Dr. Tatsuya Mima of Kyoto University), and augmenting cognition

(Dr. Yves Rossetti, Dr. Shigeru Kitazawa, and Dr. Katsumi Watanabe of The University of Tokyo). Each lecturer and speaker contributed a chapter to this book. Eight young investigators also gave 7-min presentations, and Dr. Akitoshi Ogawa of RIKEN Brain Science Institute and Dr. Satoko Koganemaru of Kyoto University included these contributions in their chapters. This book is the outcome of the conference. Consequently, it does not cover all of the research topics in the field of systems neuroscience; that said, however, we are confident that this book constitutes a solid foundation for researchers who aim to contribute scientifically to the project of helping persons with disabilities expand their range of activities.

In closing, we would like to express our profound gratitude to the NRCD executives – Dr. Tsutomu Iwaya, Dr. Fumio Eto, Dr. Masami Akai, Dr. Motoi Suwa, and Dr. Yasoichi Nakajima – and for a Grant-in-Aid from the Ministry of Health, Labour, and Welfare (Japan) for supporting both the conference and the publication of this book.

Tokorozawa   Kenji Kansaku, M.D., Ph.D.
January 2011

Contents

Contributors

Masami Akai
Department of Rehabilitation for Movement Functions, Research Institute
of National Rehabilitation Center for Persons with Disabilities (NRCD),
4-1 Namiki, Tokorozawa, Saitama 359-8555, Japan

Niels Birbaumer
Institute of Medical Psychology and Behavioral Neurobiology,
University of Tübingen, Tübingen, Germany

Ospedale san Camillo, IRCCS, Venice, Italy

Leonardo G. Cohen
Human Cortical Physiology and Stroke Neurorehabilitation Section,
National Institute of Neurological Disorders and Stroke (NINDS),
National Institutes of Health (NIH), 10 Center Drive, Bethesda,
MD 20892-1430, USA

Kazuhisa Domen
Department of Physical and Rehabilitation Medicine,
Hyogo College of Medicine, 1-1 Mukogawa-cho, Nishinomiya,
Hyogo 663-8501, Japan

Alessandro Farné
Centre de recherche en Neurosciences de Lyon, Inserm U1028,
CRNS UMR5092, ImpAct, 16 avenue Lépine, Bron, France

Université de Lyon, Université Lyon 1, Lyon, France

Hidenao Fukuyama
Human Brain Research Center, Kyoto University School of Medicine,
54 Shogoin Kawahara-cho, Sakyo-ku, Kyoto 606-8507, Japan

Sophie Jacquin-Ciourtois
Centre de recherche en Neurosciences de Lyon, Inserm U1028,
CRNS UMR5092, ImpAct, 16 avenue Lépine, Bron, France

Université de Lyon, Université Lyon 1, Lyon, France

Service de Rééducation Neurologique, Plate-forme Mouvement et Handicap,
Hôpital Henry Gabrielle, Hospices Civils de Lyon, Route de Vourles,
69230, St Genis Laval, France

Hiroyuki Kambara
Tokyo Institute of Technology, 4259-R2-15, Nagatsuta-cho, Midori-ku,
Yokohama, Kanagawa 226-8503, Japan

Kenji Kansaku
Systems Neuroscience Section, Department of Rehabilitation for Brain
Functions, Research Institute of National Rehabilitation Center for Persons
with Disabilities (NRCD), 4-1 Namiki, Tokorozawa, Saitama 359-8555, Japan

Noritaka Kawashima
Department of Rehabilitation for Movement Functions, Research Institute
of National Rehabilitation Center for Persons with Disabilities (NRCD), 4-1 Namiki,
Tokorozawa, Saitama 359-8555, Japan

Shigeru Kitazawa
Department of Neurophysiology, Juntendo University Graduate School
of Medicine, 2-1-1 Hongo, Bunkyo-ku, Tokyo 113-8421, Japan

Satoko Koganemaru
Human Brain Research Center, Kyoto University School of Medicine,
54 Shogoin Kawahara-cho, Sakyo-ku, Kyoto 606-8507, Japan

Department of Physical and Rehabilitation Medicine, Hyogo College
of Medicine, 1-1 Mukogawa-cho, Nishinomiya, Hyogo 663-8501, Japan

Yasuharu Koike
Tokyo Institute of Technology, 4259-R2-15, Nagatsuta-cho,
Midori-ku, Yokohama, Kanagawa 226-8503, Japan

JST CREST, 4-1-8 Honmachi, Kawaguchi, Saitama, Japan

Jacques Luauté
Centre de recherche en Neurosciences de Lyon, Inserm U1028,
CRNS UMR5092, ImpAct, 16 avenue Lépine, Bron, France

Université de Lyon, Université Lyon 1, Lyon, France

Service de Rééducation Neurologique, Plate-forme Mouvement
et Handicap, Hôpital Henry Gabrielle, Hospices Civils de Lyon,
Route de Vourles, 69230, St Genis Laval, France

Tatsuya Mima
Human Brain Research Center, Kyoto University School of Medicine,
54 Shogoin Kawahara-cho, Sakyo-ku, Kyoto 606-8507, Japan

Tamami Nakano
Department of Neurophysiology, Juntendo University Graduate School
of Medicine, 2-1-1 Hongo, Bunkyo-ku, Tokyo 113-8421, Japan
CREST, Japan Science and Technology Agency, Kawaguchi,
Saitama 332-0012, Japan

Kimitaka Nakazawa
Department of Rehabilitation for Movement Functions, Research Institute
of National Rehabilitation Center for Persons with Disabilities (NRCD),
4-1 Namiki, Tokorozawa, Saitama 359-8555, Japan

Toru Ogata
Department of Rehabilitation for Movement Functions, Research Institute
of National Rehabilitation Center for Persons with Disabilities (NRCD),
4-1 Namiki, Tokorozawa, Saitama 359-8555, Japan

Akitoshi Ogawa
RIKEN Brain Science Institute, 2-1 Hirosawa, Wako, Saitama 351-0198, Japan

Jacinta O'Shea
Centre for Functional Magnetic Resonance Imaging of the Brain (FMRIB),
Nuffield Department of Clinical Neurosciences, University of Oxford,
Oxford, UK

Laure Pisella
Centre de recherche en Neurosciences de Lyon, Inserm U1028,
CRNS UMR5092, ImpAct, 16 avenue Lépine, Bron, France
Université de Lyon, Université Lyon 1, Lyon, France

Patrice Revol
Centre de recherche en Neurosciences de Lyon, Inserm U1028,
CRNS UMR5092, ImpAct, 16 avenue Lépine, Bron, France
Université de Lyon, Université Lyon 1, Lyon, France
Service de Rééducation Neurologique, Plate-forme Mouvement et Handicap,
Hôpital Henry Gabrielle, Hospices Civils de Lyon, Route de Vourles,
69230, St Genis Laval, France

Gilles Rode
Centre de recherche en Neurosciences de Lyon, Inserm U1028,
CRNS UMR5092, ImpAct, 16 avenue Lépine, Bron, France
Université de Lyon, Université Lyon 1, Lyon, France
Service de Rééducation Neurologique, Plate-forme Mouvement et Handicap,
Hôpital Henry Gabrielle, Hospices Civils de Lyon, Route de Vourles,
69230, St Genis Laval, France

Yves Rossetti
Centre de recherche en Neurosciences de Lyon, Inserm U1028,
CRNS UMR5092, ImpAct, 16 avenue Lépine, Bron, France

Université de Lyon, Université Lyon 1, Lyon, France

Service de Rééducation Neurologique, Plate-forme Mouvement et Handicap,
Hôpital Henry Gabrielle, Hospices Civils de Lyon, Route de Vourles,
69230, St Genis Laval, France

Duk Shin
Tokyo Institute of Technology, 4259-R2-15, Nagatsuta-cho, Midori-ku,
Yokohama, Kanagawa 226-8503, Japan

Surjo R. Soekadar
Human Cortical Physiology and Stroke Neurorehabilitation Section,
National Institute of Neurological Disorders and Stroke (NINDS),
National Institutes of Health (NIH), 10 Center Drive, Bethesda,
MD 20892-1430, USA

Institute of Medical Psychology and Behavioral Neurobiology,
University of Tübingen, Tübingen, Germany

Katsumi Watanabe
Research Center for Advanced Science and Technology, The University of Tokyo,
4-6-1 Komaba, Meguro-ku, Tokyo 153-8904, Japan

National Institute of Advanced Industrial Science and Technology,
1-1-1 Higashi, Tsukuba, Ibaraki, Japan

Natsue Yoshimura
Tokyo Institute of Technology, 4259-R2-15, Nagatsuta-cho,
Midori-ku, Yokohama, Kanagawa 226-8503, Japan

Part I
Brain–Machine Interfaces and Neurorehabilitation

Brain–Computer Interfaces in the Rehabilitation of Stroke and Neurotrauma

Surjo R. Soekadar, Niels Birbaumer, and Leonardo G. Cohen

Abstract Paralysis after stroke or neurotrauma is among the leading causes of long term disability in adults. The development of brain–computer interface (BCI) systems that allow online classification of electric or metabolic brain activity and their translation into control signals of external devices or computers have led to two major approaches in tackling the problem of paralysis. While *assistive* BCI systems strive for continuous high-dimensional control of robotic devices or functional electric stimulation (FES) of paralyzed muscles to substitute for lost motor functions in a daily life environment (e.g. Velliste et al. 2008 [1]; Hochberg et al. 2006 [2]; Pfurtscheller et al. 2000 [3]), *restorative* BCI systems aim at normalization of neurophysiologic activity that might facilitate motor recovery (e.g. Birbaumer et al. 2007, 2009 [4, 5]; Daly et al. 2008 [6]). In order to make assistive BCI systems work in daily life, high BCI communication speed is necessary, an issue that by now can

L.G. Cohen (✉)
Human Cortical Physiology and Stroke Neurorehabilitation Section,
National Institute of Neurological Disorders and Stroke (NINDS), National Institutes
of Health (NIH), 10 Center Drive, Bethesda, MD 20892-1430, USA
e-mail: cohenl@ninds.nih.gov

S.R. Soekadar
Human Cortical Physiology and Stroke Neurorehabilitation Section,
National Institute of Neurological Disorders and Stroke (NINDS), National Institutes
of Health (NIH), 10 Center Drive, Bethesda, MD 20892-1430, USA
and
Institute of Medical Psychology and Behavioral Neurobiology, University of Tübingen,
Tübingen, Germany

N. Birbaumer
Institute of Medical Psychology and Behavioral Neurobiology, University of Tübingen,
Tübingen, Germany
and
Ospedale san Camillo, IRCCS, Venice, Italy

only be achieved by invasive recordings of brain activity (e.g. via multi-unit arrays, MUA, or electrocorticogram, ECoG). Restorative BCI systems, in contrast, were developed as training tools based on non-invasive methods such as electro- or magnetoencephalography (EEG/MEG). More recently developed approaches use real-time functional magnetic resonance imaging (rtfMRI) or near-infrared spectroscopy (NIRS). Here, we provide an overview of the current state in the development and application of assistive and restorative BCI and introduce novel approaches to improve BCI control with brain stimulation such as transcranial direct current stimulation (tDCS). The outlook of using BCI in rehabilitation of stroke and neurotrauma is discussed.

Introduction

Since the development of electroencephalographic measurements (EEG) in the early twentieth century based on Hans Berger's discovery of electric brain oscillations [7], the idea of reading out thoughts from brain activity fired the imagination of many scientists. Most recent advances in sensor technology and computational capacities led to the development of brain–computer interfaces (BCI). These systems allow direct translation of electric or metabolic brain activity into control signals of external devices or computers. While BCI systems based on classification of action potential spike trains recorded by single or multi-unit electrodes or local field potentials (LFP) recorded by electrocorticography (ECoG) require implantation (invasive BCI) [1, 8–11], well established techniques such as electroencephalography (EEG) and magnetoencephalography (MEG) allow non-invasive BCI control [12–16]. More recent developments use near-infrared-spectroscopy (NIRS) or real-time functional magnetic resonance imaging (rtfMRI) in BCI systems [17].

By creating an alternative efferent pathway of the brain, BCI were successfully used for communication [12, 18] or control of orthotic devices that would allow hemiplegic patients e.g. to grasp [19].

Stroke and neurotrauma belong to the leading causes for long-term disability worldwide and the number of affected people increases every year due to demographic change and increasing survival rates [20]. Up to 30% of all stroke victims experience very limited motor recovery and depend on assistance to manage their daily living activities [21, 22]. Enabling those patients to regain the ability to move their paralyzed limbs, respectively improving their capacity for motor behavior, could substantially improve their quality of life. While there are encouraging studies providing evidence that e.g. constrained-induced therapy (CIT) or bilateral arm training might be useful strategies for rehabilitation of stroke patients with paretic upper extremities [23, 24], there is no accepted and efficient rehabilitation strategy for severely affected stroke patients with completely paralyzed muscles, precisely those who cannot participate in common training-based rehabilitative treatments.

Assistive and Restorative BCI in Neurorehabilitation

Depending on the aim of BCI use in rehabilitation of paralysis, two major approaches can be distinguished: while *assistive* BCI systems aim at high dimensional control of robotic limbs or functional electric stimulation (FES) that specifically activate paralyzed muscles to substitute a lost motor function in daily life [1, 2, 25], *restorative* BCI aim at selective induction of use-dependent neuroplasticity to facilitate motor recovery [26–29].

These two approaches derive from different research traditions and are not necessarily related to the invasiveness of the approach: In early work of Eberhard Fetz (1969) a monkey learned, based on operant conditioning, to use cortical unit activity to deflect a lever delivering reward [30]. Two decades later, decoding of different movement directions from single neurons was achieved [31, 32]. Since then the reconstruction of complex movements from neuronal activity became possible. Firing patterns of single cells of the motor cortex [33] or parietal neuronal pools [34] in animals were remarkably successful to reconstruct movement trajectories. Monkeys learned to control cursors towards moving targets on a computer screen in a predetermined sequence by successively activating neurons in motor, premotor and parietal motor areas. In a particularly successful preparation, 32 cells were sufficient to move an artificial arm and perform skilful reaching movements after extensive training [1]. This technique enabled a monkey to feed himself. The plasticity of the cortical circuits allowed learned control of movements directly from the cellular activity even outside the primary or secondary homuncular representations of the motor cortex [9], a circumstance that supports the assumption that operant conditioning is a key factor for learning BCI control irrespective the area of recording. In an encouraging experiment Hochberg (2006) implanted densely packed microelectrode arrays of up to several hundred microelectrodes in two quadriplegic human patients [2]. Within a few training sessions, the patients learned to use LFP to move a computer cursor in several directions. This kind of BCI control with two degrees of freedom (DoF) could be used e.g. to switch on lights, a TV or to make a phone call. However, in contrast to the studies in healthy animals none of the invasive procedures allowed restoration of skilful movement in paralyzed humans. It is not clear why so far the human preparations have achieved only limited results in terms of application to activities of daily living. There are a couple of major challenges that are unsolved particularly stability, encapsulation and general safety issues [35–37]. While the primary motor cortex (M1) has the most non-ambiguous influence on the motor neurons of the upper limb, it is tightly connected with supplementary (SMA) and other non-primary motor areas [38] that are involved in the integration of complex skilled movements [39, 40]. Studies using retrograde transport tracers from the arm area of M1 in macaques showed, however, that up to 60% of all cortical projections to the spinal cord originate in pre-motor areas [41]. This indicates that complex motor behavior might not be exclusively decodable from the primary motor cortex and may in fact require multiple recording sites from various brain areas that integrate complex networks. In a very encouraging recent study, though, sufficient information could be extracted from a 4×4 mm grid with 96 silicon-based electrodes placed over M1 of a macaque to reconstruct 25 measured joint angles representing an estimated 10 DoF [42]. This electrode system (BrainGate II®) is currently investigated in a pilot human clinical trial to address reliability and safety.[1]

Studies using the less invasive approach of epidural implanted ECoG electrode grids showed that a subject could learn to control cursor movements with only a few minutes of training [43, 44]. Besides a better topographical resolution and recording bandwidth compared to non-invasive approaches [45, 46], ECoG based BCI have a better signal-to-noise ratio due to absence of electromyographic contaminations and other artifacts [47]. Recent work showed that prediction of a monkey's 3D hand trajectories and 7 DoF arm joint angles are possible with accuracy similar to recordings based on single-cell-recordings [48]. The level of DoF that can be achieved with an ECoG-grid by decoding movement associated LFP in patients with brain lesions is unclear, though, and matter of investigation.

Although not entirely impossible [49, 50], extraction and online decoding of movement trajectories from non-invasively recorded brain activity is difficult [51]. However, in contradiction to Skinner's proposal that operant and classical conditioning require involvement of the musculoskeletal system [52], voluntary control of brain oscillations is possible, opening the door to utilize this circumstance for non-invasive BCI control. The average communication rate achieved with non-invasive BCI technology in humans ranges between 5 and 25 bits/min [53], i.e. up to 25 binary (yes/no) choices can be correctly classified per minute.

Patients that are otherwise incapable to communicate, i.e. locked-in-patients suffering from amyotrophic lateral sclerosis (ALS), a disease characterized by a combined degradation of upper and lower motor neurons, can significantly benefit from non-invasive BCI use [12, 18, 54, 55]: patients are first trained to produce positive or negative slow cortical potentials (SCP) [75] upon the command of an auditory cue and after achieving more than 70% control, letters or words were presented on a computer screen. A particular letter was selected by creating SCP after its appearance [12, 14, 56, 57]. Over 40 patients with ALS at various stages of their disease were trained to use the SCP-BCI, eventually seven of these patients arrived at the locked-in-state (LIS) and were able to continue to use the BCI. All patients who began training after entering the complete locked-in-state (CLIS), however, were unable to achieve lasting BCI control [58, 59] – a finding that might be of relevance for the understanding of voluntary modulation of brain activity and BCI control.

Besides SCP, sensori-motor rhythms (SMR) are among the most investigated electro-physiologic signals used for non-invasive BCI control. The discovery of SMR dates back to the early 1950s: the observation of a local and frequency specific signal-amplitude reduction in the range of 8–13 Hz over the rolandic area during motor preparation or execution became introduced as μ-rhythm after a suggestion by Gastaut [60, 61]. Based on location, frequency and reactivity to sensory input or output, different components of the μ-rhythm were postulated [3]. The discovery of

---

[1] http://www.clinicaltrials.gov/ct2/show/NCT00912041.

event-related desynchronization (ERD) and synchronization (ERS) during motor-related activities [62] was the basis for the development of SMR-based BCI. ERD/ERS offers quantification of stimulus-locked brain activity within the time-frequency and spatial domain. It is assumed that ERD reflects extensive information processing within the sensory-motor system [63], while ERS is associated with increased synchronous idling of sensory-motor neuron networks [64]. The accessibility by cognitive manipulation makes SMR an ideal candidate to drive a BCI system. Use of SMR modulation for BCI control was extensively investigated by the Pfurtscheller group in Graz [3, 13], the Wolpaw group in Albany [65, 66] and the Birbaumer group in Tübingen [67]. In 2003, Pfurtscheller's BCI-group introduced the first SMR-based BCI that was used to enable a quadriplegic patient to control grasping through functional electrical stimulation activated by motor imagery [3].

Another well-tested BCI controller is the P300-BCI based on event-related brain potentials (ERP) by Donchin [68]. While SCP- and SMR-control is learned through visual and auditory feedback often requiring up to ten training sessions before reliable control is achieved, the P300-BCI needs no extensive training. Information rates of P300-BCI can reach 20–25 bits/min [69] but requires a very high attention level – a requirement often not met by people with neurologic or psychiatric disorders.

Most recently also a BOLD-signal based rtfMRI-BCI has been introduced [70–73]. In 2003 Weiskopf et al. [70] proposed that the development of fMRI-BCIs might be a powerful tool in the treatment of various disorders and diseases. It was shown that intracortical activity is highly correlated with local blood flow change and the BOLD signal [74] and that volitional regulation of BOLD activity in cortical and sub-cortical areas such as amygdala, anterior cingulate, insula and parahippocampal gyrus was associated with changes of connectivity between those areas [73]. DeCharms et al. [72] demonstrated that use of a real-time fMRI-BCI can affect pain perception.

In addition to the fMRI-BCI approach, near infrared spectroscopy (NIRS) is also a non-invasive technique based on measuring metabolic changes of the brain. Using multiple pairs or channels of light sources and light detectors operating at two or more discrete wavelengths at near infrared range (700–1,000 nm) cerebral oxygenation and blood flow of particular regions of the cortical surface can be determined. The degree of increase in regional cerebral blood flow (rCBF) exceeds that of increase in regional cerebral oxygen metabolic rate (rCMRO$_2$) resulting in a decrease in deoxygenated hemoglobin in venous blood during higher oxygen demand. Therefore, an increase in total hemoglobin and oxygenated hemoglobin with a decrease in deoxygenated hemoglobin can be measured in activated active brain areas. The recent development of portable systems makes NIRS a promising tool in non-invasive BCI research [17, 28].

In contrast to this work aiming at assistive appliance of invasive and non-invasive BCI technology, the development of *restorative* BCI systems is tightly associated with the development and successes of neurofeedback (NF) and its use to purposefully up-regulate or down-regulate brain activity – a quality that showed to have some beneficial effect in the treatment of various neurological and psychiatric disorders associated with neurophysiologic abnormalities [5]. In NF subjects receive visual or auditory on-line feedback of their brain activity and are asked to voluntarily modify e.g. a particular type of brainwave [5]. The feedback contains the information on the degree of success in controlling the signal and delivers the reward for correct modification. NF was successfully used in the treatment of epilepsy [76, 77], ADHD [78–80], chronic pain syndrome [81] and complete paralysis after stroke [3].

Stroke can be associated with extensive neuroplastic changes on the synaptic, neuronal and circuit level. Besides new synapses strengthening and rewiring [82] as a consequence of long-term potentiation (LTP) or long-term depression (LTD), dendritic sprouting, extensive peri-infarct reorganization and changes of activity patterns in remote cortical regions [83] including interhemispheric inhibition [84–87] were described.

Various interventions that aim at modulation of neuroplasticity, such as reduction of somatosensory input from the intact hand [88] or increase from the affected hand [89], neuropharmacologic strategies influencing dopaminergic or adrenergic systems [90], mental training such as motor-imagery training [91–93] and non-invasive brain stimulation [93–96] showed to have beneficial effects on motor function after stroke.

It was shown that the ability to desynchronize the affected hemisphere in the SMR-range during the acute and sub-acute phase of stroke correlates with clinical motor outcome [97]. A finding that is consistent with fMRI studies performed in stroke patients that suggested an association of increased activity in the ipsilesional primary motor cortex and functional recovery while involvement of the contrale-sional motor cortex during movements of the affected hand was associated with poor motor recovery [98, 99].

Following these lines, a restorative BCI is based on two hypotheses: (1) By inducing CNS plasticity that produces more normal activation (e.g. in terms of lat-eralization), normal motor function will be restored. (2) Contingent sensory input given as reward to a specific activation pattern in the motor system induces CNS plasticity that facilitates restoration of normal motor control, potentially through rewiring and synaptic strengthening of weakened or previously inhibited motor networks.

As an important step for further development of SMR-based assistive and restor-ative BCI systems, a study was conducted by Buch et al. (2008) [19] to evaluate whether patients with chronic stroke would be able to learn to modulate μ-rhythm. Eight patients with chronic hand plegia resulting from stroke participated in 13–22 BCI training sessions to learn voluntary control of their μ-rhythm amplitude origi-nating in the sensori-motor areas of the cortex. Diagnostic MRIs revealed single, unilateral subcortical, cortical or mixed lesions in the participating patients. Patients had no residual finger extension function. Before the actual training, the patients had to imagine several distinct movements of the upper and lower extremity as well as the tongue. While doing this, the ipsilesional area with the strongest oscillatory MEG response in the μ-range was identified. Based on the area's location, three MEG sensors were selected for BCI control. During the training, μ-desynchroniza-tion was translated in cursor-movements on a screen. After approximately 4 s of either up or down regulation, the affected hand was either opened or closed by a hand-orthosis affixed to the participant's paralyzed fingers. At the end of the training, SMR control was associated with increased range and specificity of μ-rhythm modulation as recorded from sensors overlying central ipsilesional (four patients) or contralesional (two patients) regions. However, two patients were unable to gain BCI control. One patient started with high success rates of BCI control (approximately 85%) at the beginning of the training and did not improve much further. This study demonstrated for the first time that most patients with chronic stroke, even with complete hand paralysis, could learn to control SMR-based BCI-systems.

However, the applied BCI training was not associated with notable clinical improvement. Up to 1 h of BCI training per day for 2–3 weeks might be insufficient to induce relevant motor recovery in patients with chronic paralysis after stroke. Other reasons might have been the limited translation of BCI-associated movements into daily-life activities ("transfer package") [100] and the delay of BCI-driven somato-sensory input, which resulted in low temporal contingence of brain activation and sensory feedback. Larger clinical studies using BCI systems that couples highly specific temporo-spatial brain activation patterns online with contingent sensory feedback might help to elucidate the viability of SMR-based BCI systems for restoration of paralysis. Unpublished data by Buch et al. indicate that fronto-parietal connectivity plays a key-role for successful SMR-based BCI learning after stroke [101].

Most recently Broetz et al. (2010) [26] published a proof-of-principle study on the combination of BCI training and goal-directed physical therapy in chronic stroke. A 67-year-old hemiplegic patient who suffered from a subcortical bleeding received three blocks of BCI training coupled with goal-directed physical therapy over the course of 12 months. Before the training he had no active finger movements, depended on assistance for personal hygiene and dressing and used a wheelchair for all distances greater than half a mile. Each BCI training block consisted of daily SMR-based BCI training over 30 days. For the first BCI training block a 275-sensor MEG was used to translate motor imagery associated SMR-modulation on the affected hemisphere into opening or closing of the paralyzed hand [25]. The second and third training block was based on EEG-recordings. Goal-directed physical therapy was continued throughout the 12 months. Arm motor function as well as gait (using Fugl-Meyer Assessment, FMA, Wolf Motor Function Test, WMFT, and Ashworth Scale) and brain reorganization was assessed repeatedly during the study. After 1 year, FMA, WMFT and Ashworth scores improved by a mean of 46.6%. The patient was able to extend his fingers and to open his affected hand to grasp. He regularly walked distances over half a mile and did not use the wheelchair anymore. Analysis of spectral amplitudes in MEG data reflecting cortical activity revealed a significantly stronger SMR-desynchronization during motor imagery and motor execution on the affected hemisphere.

A multimodal neuroimaging approach based on fMRI and diffusion tensor imaging (DTI) was used to further examine neuroplastic changes in parallel with the longitudinal clinical evaluation [27]. Psycho-physiological interaction (PPI) analysis was used to assess functional connectivity and showed that activity of ipsilesional pre-motor cortex (PMC) positively co-varied with ipsilesional primary and secondary sensorimotor areas across all measurements. Cortico-spinal tract (CST) integrity was estimated based on DTI analysis and tractography showing a significant decrease of detectable ipsilesional CST fibers by 98% in the anterior part of the posterior capsula interna, while leaving evidence of most preserved fibers in the anterior part of the internal capsule. It was proposed that the anterior fibers of the CST originating from anterior parts of the primary motor cortex (M1) or PMC might constitute the anatomical pre-requisite for the observed clinical improvement. Analysis of fMRI data revealed increased activity in the ipsilesional dorsal premotor region and supplementary motor areas at the end of the last BCI training block, and a significant increase in fractional anisotropy (FA) reflecting white matter microstructure's integrity in the affected CST. This proof-of-principle study provided encouraging data that SMR-based BCI training coupled with goal-directed physiotherapy might induce beneficial used-dependent plasticity in the perilesional areas facilitating motor recovery.

Another study by Ang and colleagues (2010) [102] compared two groups of sub-acute and chronic stroke patients (1–35 months after stroke) with predominantly sub-cortical brain lesions (80%) who received either a standardized (n = 10) or BCI-driven (n = 8) robotic rehabilitation, which was applied over 12 sessions within 4 weeks. During the standardized robotic rehabilitation training the participant's affected arm was strapped to a robotic device (MIT-Manus). Participants were instructed to move their paretic hand according to a visually presented goal on a screen in front of them. If the subject could not perform the movement on their own, the robot would assist and actively guide the subject's arm towards the goal. In the BCI group, assistive movements were only performed if SMR-ERD was detectable over the affected hemisphere during the trial. Both groups were clinically evaluated using FMA before and after the training. FMA scores ranged between 4 and 61 points (mean 29.7 +/− 17.7) before training onset. Correcting for age and gender among the subjects with positive gain, the BCI group improved more and yielded a higher gain 2-month post-rehabilitation compared to the group that received standardized robotic rehabilitation. Besides limitations of this study due to the small sample size as well as heterogeneity of the groups regarding lesion site, age and time after stroke, it provided supportive data on the potential benefit of BCI training in the context of stroke rehabilitation.

A study performed by Daly et al. (2009) [29] combined an EEG-BCI training with FES of paralyzed finger muscles. A 43-year-old 10-months post-stroke patient with a lesion affecting the left cortical and sub-cortical regions of the frontal and parietal lobe underwent nine sessions of BCI-FES training within 3 weeks. During the training the patient had to either imagine or attempt finger movements on the affected side in alternation with attempted relaxation. Before the training, the patient could not actively extent the affected index finger. Sustained motor-related ERD was translated in activation of the FES device. During the BCI sessions the patient achieved good BCI control (over 88% in eight of nine sessions for attempted movement) and regained 26 degrees of volitional isolated index finger extension after session nine.

While all these reports are encouraging, larger controlled clinical studies are necessary to further evaluate the potential role of non-invasive assistive and restorative BCI technology in the rehabilitation of stroke and neurotrauma. Anatomical and functional pre-requisites for successful SMR-based BCI learning and mechanisms underlying clinical improvements need to be identified and well characterized.

As some of the stroke patients did not gain SMR-based BCI control, strategies to improve BCI learning would be of particular importance. In this context, techniques that can be used to modulate cortical plasticity such as transcranial direct current stimulation (tDCS) or transcranial magnetic stimulation (TMS) could be helpful tools to develop better BCI training protocols in patient groups.

Improving BCI Performance with Brain Stimulation

It was shown that transcranial direct current stimulation (tDCS), a non-invasive and well-tolerated method based on application of weak direct currents (e.g. 1 mA delivered for 20 min) through saline-soaked sponges attached to the head, can induce polarity specific changes of excitability in M1 [103] and, thus, enhance activity within M1. Further studies suggested that tDCS over M1 could be used to improve motor learning and consolidation [104–106]. After stroke, modulation of M1 excitability of the affected hemisphere by anodal tDCS was associated with motor function improvements of the paretic hand [94, 107]. A pilot study on combined tDCS and robot-assisted arm training by Hesse et al. (2007) [94] indicated beneficial effects on motor function (assessed by FMA) and aphasia in several participants.

Another non-invasive and well-established technique to modulate brain excitability is transcranial magnetic stimulation (TMS). In TMS a magnetic field is used to induce a small electric current that can lead to depolarization of cortical neurons. Depending on the intensity and frequency of stimulation, TMS can have lasting effects on the excitability of the brain when delivered repetitively (rTMS). Also, based on the finding that rTMS can elicit long lasting excitatory or inhibitory effects, use of rTMS as a therapeutic tool in neurological and psychiatric disorders, such as depression [108], chronic pain [109], epilepsy [110] or movement disorders [111] became investigated. In stroke, low-frequency (inhibitory) rTMS was used to reduce cortical excitability in the unaffected primary motor cortex and resulted in transient improvements of motor function [112–114]. Targeting the affected hemisphere of stroke patients with high-frequency (excitatory) rTMS, motor function improvements were reported [115, 116].

As SMR-related ERD can be interpreted as an electrophysiological correlate of cortical activation [117], anodal tDCS or high-frequency rTMS applied to the affected motor cortex might be a useful tool to improve ERD-dependent BCI performance in stroke patients and hence enhance practicability of assistive and restorative BCI systems.

Prospects of BCI Applications in Stroke and Neurotrauma

The development of assistive and restorative BCI technology for rehabilitation of stroke or neurotrauma is an exciting emerging field that yields notable potential to improve quality of life for many affected people. So far, only few studies on application of invasive or non-invasive BCI technology in patients with stroke or neurotrauma are available [19, 26, 29, 102]. Mechanisms underlying voluntary SMR-modulation for BCI control are not well understood. Optimal settings and algorithms for BCI training protocols in patients with brain lesions are unknown. Therefore, studies based on MEG recordings for BCI control are of particular importance as MEG allows precise and relatively artifact-free post-hoc analysis of cortical activity patterns.

EEG-based BCI systems have the best potential for widespread clinical use. However, preparation time and sensitivity to muscle artifacts limit their practicability. The development of dry-electrode-systems with portable amplifiers offers a promising perspective. In this context the combination with FES systems and simultaneous electric brain stimulation represents a propitious vista for both, assistive and restorative BCI systems. While costly at present, BCI systems based on NIRS might become an attractive alternative to EEG.

New concepts for innovative BCI approaches based on measures that are currently too complex for online applications, such as dual-core beamforming [118] that allow identification of simultaneously active correlated networks, might become feasible once required computational capacities are available.

More and larger clinical studies are needed to develop optimal protocols for both, assistive and restorative BCI applications. Due to the heterogeneity of patient populations, multimodal approaches to evaluate subject specific characteristics in terms of anatomy and function including e.g. fMRI, DTI, MEG and diagnostic TMS are an important pre-requisite for a better understanding of BCI related neuroplasticity and might help to develop new strategies for BCI use in neurorehabilitation.

Conclusion

Assistive and restorative BCI technology might be a powerful tool to improve rehabilitation strategies in patients with brain lesions and severe motor paralysis, such as stroke or traumatic brain injury.

Acknowledgements This contribution was supported by the NINDS intramural research program of the National Institutes of Health (NIH), the Deutsche Forschungsgemeinschaft (DFG) and the German Ministry of Education and Research (BMBF, 01GQ0831).

References

1. Velliste M, Perel S, Spalding MC, Whitford AS, Schwartz AB (2008) Cortical control of a prosthetic arm for self-feeding. Nature 453:1098–1101
2. Hochberg LR, Serruya MD, Friehs GM, Mukand JA, Saleh M, Caplan AH, Branner A, Chen D, Penn RD, Donoghue JP (2006) Neural ensemble control of prosthetic devices by a human with tetraplegia. Nature 442:164–171

3. Pfurtscheller G, Guger C, Muller G, Krausz G, Neuper C (2000) Brain oscillations control hand orthosis in a tetraplegic. Neurosci Lett 292:211–214
4. Birbaumer N, Cohen LG (2007) Brain–computer interfaces: communication and restoration of movement in paralysis. J Physiol 579:621–636
5. Birbaumer N, Ramos Murguialday A, Weber C, Montoya P (2009) Neurofeedback and brain–computer interface clinical applications. Int Rev Neurobiol 86:107–117
6. Daly JJ, Wolpaw JR (2008) Brain–computer interfaces in neurological rehabilitation. Lancet Neurol 7:1032–1043
7. Berger H (1929) Ueber das Elektrenkephalogramm des Menschen. Archiv für Psychiatrie und Nervenkrankheiten 87:527–570
8. Serruya MD, Hatsopoulos NG, Paninski L, Fellows MR, Donoghue JP (2002) Instant neural control of a movement signal. Nature 416:141–142
9. Taylor DM, Tillery SI, Schwartz AB (2002) Direct cortical control of 3D neuroprosthetic devices. Science 296:1829–1832
10. Carmena JM, Lebedev MA, Crist RA, O'Doherty JA, Santucci DM, Dimitrov DF, Patil PG, Henriquez CS, Nicolelis MAL (2003) Learning to control a brain–machine interface for reaching and grasping by primates. PLoS Biol 1:1–16
11. Donoghue JP, Nurmikko A, Black M, Hochberg LR (2007) Assistive technology and robotic control using motor cortex ensemble-based neural interface systems in humans with tetraplegia. J Physiol 579:603–611
12. Birbaumer N, Ghanayim N, Hinterberger T, Iversen I, Kotchoubey B, Kubler A, Perelmouter J, Taub E, Flor H (1999) A spelling device for the paralyzed. Nature 398:297–298
13. Pfurtscheller G, Graimann B, Huggins JE, Levine SP (2004) Brain–computer communication based on the dynamics of brain oscillations. Suppl Clin Neurophysiol 57:583–591
14. Wolpaw JR, Birbaumer N, McFarland DJ, Pfurtscheller G, Vaughan TM (2002) Brain–computer interfaces for communication and control. Clin Neurophysiol 113:767–791
15. McFarland DJ, Krusienski DJ, Sarnacki WA, Wolpaw JR (2008) Emulation of computer mouse control with a noninvasive brain–computer interface. J Neural Eng 5:101–110
16. Blankertz B, Dornhege G, Krauledat M, Muller KR, Curio G (2007) The non-invasive Berlin brain–computer interface: fast acquisition of effective performance in untrained subjects. Neuroimage 37:539–550
17. Sitaram R, Caria A, Birbaumer N (2009) Hemodynamic brain–computer interfaces for communication and rehabilitation. Neural Netw 22:1320–1328
18. Kübler A, Nijboer F, Mellinger J, Vaughan TM, Pawelzik H, Schalk G, McFarland DJ, Birbaumer N, Wolpaw JR (2005) Patients with ALS can use sensorimotor rhythms to operate a brain–computer interface. Neurology 64:1775–1777
19. Buch E, Weber C, Cohen LG, Braun C, Dimyan MA, Ard T, Mellinger J, Caria A, Soekadar S, Fourkas A, Birbaumer N (2008) Think to move: a neuromagnetic brain–computer interface (BCI) system for chronic stroke. Stroke 39:910–917
20. Organization WH (2003) The World Health report: shaping the future. World Health Organization, Geneva, p 2003
21. Kwakkel G, Kollen BJ, van der Grond J, Prevo AJ (2003) Probability of regaining dexterity in the flaccid upper limb: impact of severity of paresis and time since onset in acute stroke. Stroke 34:2181–2186
22. Rosamond W, Flegal K, Furie K, Go A, Greenlund K, Haase N, Hailpern SM, Ho M, Howard V, Kissela B, Kittner S, Lloyd-Jones D, McDermott M, Meigs J, Moy C, Nichol G, O'Donnell C, Roger V, Sorlie P, Steinberger J, Thom T, Wilson M, Hong Y (2008) Heart disease and stroke statistics – 2008 update: a report from the American Heart Association Statistics Committee and Stroke Statistics Subcommittee. Circulation 117:e25–e146
23. Wolf SL, Winstein CJ, Miller JP, Taub E, Uswatte G, Morris D, Giuliani C, Light KE, Nichols-Larsen D, EXCITE Investigators (2006) Effect of constraint-induced movement therapy on upper extremity function 3 to 9 months after stroke – the EXCITE randomized clinical trial. JAMA 296:2095–2104

24. Luft AR, McCombe-Waller S, Whitall J, Forrester LW, Macko R, Sorkin JD, Schulz JB, Goldberg AP, Hanley DF (2004) Repetitive bilateral arm training and motor cortex activation in chronic stroke: a randomized controlled trial. JAMA 292:1853–1861

25. Pfurtscheller G, Müller GR, Pfurtscheller J, Gerner HJ, Rupp R (2003) 'Thought' – control of functional electrical stimulation to restore hand grasp in a patient with tetraplegia. Neurosci Lett 351:33–36

26. Broetz D, Braun C, Weber C, Soekadar SR, Caria A, Birbaumer N (2010) Combination of brain–computer interface training and goal-directed physical therapy in chronic stroke: a case report. Neurorehabil Neural Repair 24:674–679

27. Caria A, Weber C, Brötz D, Ramos A, Ticini LF, Gharabaghi A, Braun C, Birbaumer N (2010) Chronic stroke recovery after combined BCI training and physiotherapy: A case report. Psychophysiology 48:578–582

28. Nagaoka T, Sakatani K, Awano T, Yokose N, Hoshino T, Murata Y, Katayama Y, Ishikawa A, Eda H (2010) Development of a new rehabilitation system based on a brain–computer interface using near-infrared spectroscopy. Adv Exp Med Biol 662:497–503

29. Daly JJ, Cheng R, Rogers J, Litinas K, Hrovat K, Dohring M (2009) Feasibility of a new application of noninvasive brain computer interface (BCI): a case study of training for recovery of volitional motor control after stroke. J Neurol Phys Ther 33:203–211

30. Fetz EE (1969) Operant conditioning of cortical unit activity. Science 163:955–958

31. Georgopoulos AP, Schwartz AB, Kettner RE (1986) Neuronal population coding of movement direction. Science 233:1416–1419

32. Georgopoulos AP, Lurito JT, Petrides M, Schwartz AB, Massey JT (1989) Mental rotation of the neuronal population vector. Science 243:234–236

33. Nicolelis MA (2003) Brain–machine interfaces to restore motor function and probe neural circuits. Nat Rev Neurosci 4:417–422

34. Scherberger H, Jarvis MR, Andersen RA (2005) Cortical local field potentials encodes movement intentions in the posterior parietal cortex. Neuron 46:347–354

35. Dickey AS, Suminski A, Amit Y, Hatsopoulos NG (2009) Single-unit stability using chronically implanted multielectrode arrays. J Neurophysiol 102:1331–1339

36. Rousche PJ, Normann RA (1998) Chronic recording capability of the Utah intracortical electrode array in cat sensory cortex. J Neurosci Methods 82:1–15

37. Fountas KN, Smith JR (2007) Subdural electrode-associated complications: a 20-year experience. Stereotact Funct Neurosurg 85:264–272

38. Penfield W, Welch K (1951) The supplementary motor area of the cerebral cortex; a clinical and experimental study. AMA Arch Neurol Psychiatry 66:289–317

39. Fulton JF (1934) A note on the definition of the motor and premotor areas. Brain 57:311–316

40. Fulton JF (1935) Definition of the 'motor' and 'premotor' areas. Brain 58:311–316

41. Dum RP, Strick PL (1991) The origin of corticospinal projections from the premotor areas in the frontal lobe. J Neurosci 11:667–689

42. Vargas-Irwin CE, Shakhnarovich G, Yadollahpour P, Mislow JM, Black MJ, Donoghue JP (2010) Decoding complete reach and grasp actions from local primary motor cortex populations. J Neurosci 30:9659–9669

43. Schalk G, Miller KJ, Anderson NR, Wilson JA, Smyth MD, Ojemann JG, Moran DW, Wolpaw JR, Leuthardt EC (2008) Two-dimensional movement control using electrocorticographic signals in humans. J Neural Eng 5:75–84

44. Leuthardt EC, Schalk G, Wolpaw JR, Ojemann JG, Moran DW (2004) A brain–computer interface using electrocorticographic signals in humans. J Neural Eng 1:63–71

45. Freeman WJ, Rogers LJ, Holmes MD, Silbergeld DL (2000) Spatial spectral analysis of human electrocorticograms including the alpha and gamma bands. J Neurosci Methods 95:111–121

46. Staba RJ, Wilson CL, Bragin A, Fried I, Engel J Jr (2002) Quantitative analysis of high-frequency oscillations (80–500 Hz) recorded in human epileptic hippocampus and entorhinal cortex. J Neurophysiol 88:1743–1752

47. Ball T, Kern M, Mutschler I, Aertsen A, Schulze-Bonhage A (2009) Signal quality of simultaneously recorded invasive and non-invasive EEG. Neuroimage 46:708–716
48. Chao ZC, Nagasaka Y, Fujii N (2010) Long-term asynchronous decoding of arm motion using electrocorticographic signals in monkeys. Front Neuroeng 3:3
49. Bradberry TJ, Gentili RJ, Contreras-Vidal JL (2010) Reconstructing three-dimensional hand movements from noninvasive electroencephalographic signals. J Neurosci 30:3432–3437
50. Waldert S, Preissl H, Demandt E, Braun C, Birbaumer N, Aertsen A, Mehring C (2008) Hand movement direction decoded from MEG and EEG. J Neurosci 28:1000–1008
51. Lebedev MA, Nicolelis MA (2006) Brain–machine interfaces: past, present and future. Trends Neurosci 29:536–546
52. Skinner F (1953) Science and human behavior. Macmillan, New York
53. Wolpaw JR, Birbaumer N, Heetderks WJ, McFarland DJ, Peckham PH, Schalk G, Donchin E, Quatrano LA, Robinson CJ, Vaughan TM (2000) Brain–computer interface technology: a review of the first international meeting. IEEE Trans Rehabil Eng 8:164–173
54. Kübler A, Kotchoubey B, Kaiser J, Wolpaw J, Birbaumer N (2001) Brain–computer communication: unlocking the locked-in. Psychol Bull 127:358–375
55. Birbaumer N (2006) Breaking the silence: brain–computer interfaces (BCI) for communication and motor control. Psychophysiology 43:517–532
56. Birbaumer N, Hinterberger T, Kübler A, Neumann N (2003) The thought-translation device (TTD): neurobehavioral mechanisms and clinical outcome. IEEE Trans Neural Syst Rehabil Eng 11:120–123
57. Perelmouter J, Birbaumer N (2000) A binary spelling interface with random errors. IEEE Trans Rehabil Eng 8:227–232
58. Hinterberger T, Veit R, Wilhelm B, Weiskopf N, Vatine JJ, Birbaumer N (2005) Neuronal mechanisms underlying control of a brain–computer-interface. Eur J Neurosci 21:3169–3181
59. Wilhelm B, Jordan M, Birbaumer N (2006) Communication in locked-in syndrome: effects of imagery on salivary pH. Neurology 67:534–535
60. Gastaut H, Terzian H, Gastaut Y (1952) Study of a little electroencephalographic activity: rolandic arched rhythm. Mars Med 89:296–310
61. Howe RC, Sterman MB (1972) Cortical–subcortical EEG correlates of suppressed motor behavior during sleep and waking in the cat. J Electroencephalogr Clin Neurophysiol 32:681–695
62. Pfurtscheller G, Aranibar A (1979) Evaluation of event-related desynchronization (ERD) preceding and following self-paced movement. Electroencephgr Clin Neurophysiol 46:138–146
63. Leocani L, Toro C, Zhuang P, Gerloff C, Hallet M (2001) Event-related desynchronization in reaction time paradigms: a comparison with event-related potentials and corticospinal excitability. Clin Neurophysiol 112:923–930
64. Pfurtscheller G, Stancák A Jr, Neuper C (1996) Event-related synchronization (ERS) in the alpha band – an electrophysiological correlate of cortical idling: a review. Int J Psychophysiol 24:39–46
65. Wolpaw JR, McFarland DJ (2004) Control of a two-dimensional movement signal by a non-invasive brain–computer interface in humans. Proc Natl Acad Sci USA 101:17849–17854
66. Wolpaw JR (2007) Brain–computer interfaces as new brain output pathways. J Physiol 579:613–619
67. Mellinger J, Schalk G, Braun C, Preissl H, Rosenstiel W, Birbaumer N, Kübler A (2007) An MEG-based brain–computer interface (BCI). Neuroimage 36:581–593
68. Farwell LA, Donchin E (1988) Talking off the top of your head: toward a mental prosthesis utilizing event-related brain potentials. Electroencephalogr Clin Neurophysiol 70:510–523
69. Lenhardt A, Kaper M, Ritter HJ (2008) An adaptive P300-based online brain–computer interface. IEEE Trans Neural Syst Rehabil Eng 16:121–130
70. Weiskopf N, Veit R, Erb M, Mathiak K, Grodd W, Goebel R, Birbaumer N (2003) Physiological self-regulation of regional brain activity using real-time functional magnetic resonance imaging (fMRI): methodology and exemplary data. NeuroImage 19:577–586

71. Yoo SS, Fairneny T, Chen NK, Choo SE, Panych LP, Park H, Lee SY, Jolesz FA (2004) Brain–computer interface using fMRI: spatial navigation by thoughts. Neuroreport 15:1591–1595
72. DeCharms RC, Maeda F, Glover GH, Ludlow D, Pauly JM, Soneji D, Gabrieli JD, Mackey SC (2005) Control over brain activation and pain learned by using real-time functional MRI. Proc Natl Acad Sci USA 102:18626–18631
73. Caria A, Veit R, Sitaram R, Lotze M, Weiskopf N, Grodd W, Birbaumer N (2007) Regulation of anterior insular cortex activity using real-time fMRI. NeuroImage 35:1238–1246
74. Logothetis N, Pauls J, Augath M, Trinath T, Oeltermann A (2001) Neurophysiological investigation of the basis of the fMRI signal. Nature 412:150–157
75. Elbert T, Rockstroh B, Lutzenberger W, Birbaumer N (1984) Self-regulation of the brain and behavior. Springer, New York
76. Seifert AR, Lubar JF (1975) Reduction of epileptic seizures through EEG biofeedback training. Biol Psychol 3:157–184
77. Kotchoubey B, Strehl U, Uhlmann C, Holzapfel S, König M, Fröscher W, Blankenhorn V, Birbaumer N (2001) Modification of slow cortical potentials in patients with refractory epilepsy: a controlled outcome study. Epilepsia 42:406–416
78. Birbaumer N, Elbert T, Rockstroh B, Lutzenberger W (1986) Biofeedback of slow cortical potentials in attentional disorders. In: McCallum WC, Zappoli R, Denoth F (eds) Cerebral psychophysiology: studies in event-related potentials. Elsevier, Amsterdam
79. Strehl U, Leins U, Goth G, Klinger C, Hinterberger T, Birbaumer N (2006) Self-regulation of slow cortical potentials: a new treatment for children with attention-deficit/hyperactivity disorder. Pediatrics 118:1530–1540
80. Fuchs T, Birbaumer N, Lutzenberger W, Gruzelier JH, Kaiser J (2003) Neurofeedback training for attention-deficit/hyperactivity disorder in children: a comparison with methylphenidate. Appl Psychophysiol Biofeedback 28:1–12
81. Lotze M, Grodd W, Birbaumer N, Erb M, Huse E, Flor H (1999) Does use of a myoelectric prosthesis prevent cortical reorganization and phantom limb pain? Nat Neurosci 2:501–502
82. Chklovskii DB, Mel BW, Svoboda K (2004) Cortical rewiring and information storage. Nature 431:782–788
83. Frost SB, Barbay S, Friel KM, Plautz EJ, Nudo RJ (2003) Reorganization of remote cortical regions after ischemic brain injury: a potential substrate for stroke recovery. J Neurophysiol 89:3205–3214
84. Murase N, Duque J, Mazzocchio R, Cohen LG (2004) Influence of interhemispheric interactions on motor function in chronic stroke. Ann Neurol 55:400–409
85. Duque J, Hummel F, Celnik P, Murase N, Mazzocchio R, Cohen LG (2005) Transcallosal inhibition in chronic subcortical stroke. Neuroimage 28:940–946
86. Grefkes C, Nowak DA, Eickhoff SB, Dafotakis M, Küst J, Karbe H, Fink GR (2008) Cortical connectivity after subcortical stroke assessed with functional magnetic resonance imaging. Ann Neurol 63:236–246
87. Harris-Love ML, Perez MA, Chen R, Cohen LG (2007) Interhemispheric inhibition in distal and proximal arm representations in the primary motor cortex. J Neurophysiol 97:2511–2515
88. Floel A, Nagorsen U, Werhahn KJ, Ravindran S, Birbaumer N, Knecht S, Cohen LG (2004) Influence of somatosensory input on motor function in patients with chronic stroke. Ann Neurol 56:206–212
89. Conforto AB, Kaelin-Lang A, Cohen LG (2002) Increase in hand muscle strength of stroke patients after somatosensory stimulation. Ann Neurol 51:122–125
90. Scheidtmann K (2004) Advances in adjuvant pharmacotherapy for motor rehabilitation: effects of levodopa. Restor Neurol Neurosci 22:393–398
91. Liu KP, Chan CC, Wong RS, Kwan IW, Yau CS, Li LS, Lee TM (2009) A randomized controlled trial of mental imagery augment generalization of learning in acute poststroke patients. Stroke 40:2222–2225

92. Malouin F, Richards CL, Doyon J, Desrosiers J, Belleville S (2004) Training mobility tasks after stroke with combined mental and physical practice: a feasibility study. Neurorehabil Neural Repair 18:66–75

93. Page SJ, Levine P, Leonard A (2007) Mental practice in chronic stroke: results of a randomized, placebo-controlled trial. Stroke 38:1293–1297

94. Hummel F, Celnik P, Giraux P, Floel A, Wu WH, Gerloff C, Cohen LG (2005) Effects of non-invasive cortical stimulation on skilled motor function in chronic stroke. Brain 128:490–499

95. Hesse S, Werner C, Schonhardt EM, Bardeleben A, Jenrich W, Kirker SG (2007) Combined transcranial direct current stimulation and robot-assisted arm training in subacute stroke patients: a pilot study. Restor Neurol Neurosci 25:9–15

96. Takeuchi N, Chuma T, Matsuo Y, Watanabe I, Ikoma K (2005) Repetitive transcranial magnetic stimulation of contralesional primary motor cortex improves hand function after stroke. Stroke 36:2681–2686

97. Platz T, Kim IH, Engel U, Kieselbach A, Mauritz KH (2002) Brain activation pattern as assessed with multi-modal EEG analysis predict motor recovery among stroke patients with mild arm paresis who receive the arm ability training. Restor Neurol Neurosci 20:21–35

98. Calautti C, Naccarato M, Jones PS, Sharma N, Day DD, Carpenter AT, Bullmore ET, Warburton EA, Baron JC (2007) The relationship between motor deficit and hemisphere activation balance after stroke: a 3 T fMRI study. Neuroimage 34:322–331

99. Ward NS, Cohen LG (2004) Mechanisms underlying recovery of motor function after stroke. Arch Neurol 61:1844–1848

100. Taub E, Uswatte G, Mark VW, Morris DM (2006) The learned nonuse phenomenon: implications for rehabilitation. Eura Medicophys 42:241–256

101. Buch ER, Fourkas AD, Weber C, Birbaumer N, Cohen LG (2010) Anatomical parieto-frontal connectivity predicts performance gains in μ rhythm-based brain–computer interface (BCI) training in chronic stroke. SFN 2010, San Diego, 493.6/FFF19

102. Ang KK, Guan C, Chua KS, Ang BT, Kuah C, Wang C, Phua KS, Chin ZY, Zhang H (2010) Clinical study of neurorehabilitation in stroke using EEG-based motor imagery brain–computer interface with robotic feedback. Conf Proc IEEE Eng Med Biol Soc 1:5549–5552

103. Nitsche MA, Paulus W (2000) Excitability changes induced in the human motor cortex by weak transcranial direct current stimulation. J Physiol 527:633–639

104. Nitsche MA, Schauenburg A, Lang N, Liebetanz D, Exner C, Paulus W, Tergau F (2003) Facilitation of implicit motor learning by weak transcranial direct current stimulation of the primary motor cortex in the human. J Cognit Neurosci 15:619–626

105. Reis J, Schambra HM, Cohen LG, Buch ER, Fritsch B, Zarahn E, Celnik PA, Krakauer JW (2009) Noninvasive cortical stimulation enhances motor skill acquisition over multiple days through an effect on consolidation. Proc Natl Acad Sci USA 106:1590–1595

106. Antal A, Nitsche MA, Kincses TZ, Kruse W, Hoffmann KP, Paulus W (2004) Facilitation of visuo-motor learning by transcranial direct current stimulation of the motor and extrastriate visual areas in humans. Eur J Neurosci 19:2888–2892

107. Boggio PS, Nunes A, Rigonatti SP, Nitsche MA, Pascual-Leone A, Fregni F (2007) Repeated sessions of noninvasive brain DC stimulation is associated with motor function improvement in stroke patients. Restor Neurol Neurosci 25:123–129

108. Miniussi C, Bonato C, Bignotti S, Gazzoli A, Gennarelli M, Pasqualetti P, Tura GB, Ventriglia M, Rossini PM (2005) Repetitive transcranial magnetic simulation (rTMS) at high and low frequency: an efficacious therapy for major drug-resistant depression? Clin Neurophysiol 116:1062–1071

109. Lefaucheur JP (2004) Transcranial magnetic stimulation in the management of pain. Clin Neurophysiol (Suppl) 57:737–748

110. Theodore WH (2003) Transcranial magnetic stimulation in epilepsy. Epilepsy Curr 3:191–197

111. Fregni F, Simon DK, Wu A, Pascual-Leone A (2005) Non-invasive brain stimulation for Parkinson's disease: a systematic review and meta-analysis of the literature. J Neurol Neurosurg Psychiatry 76:1614–1623

112. Mansur CG, Fregni F, Boggio PS, Riberto M, Gallucci-Neto J, Santos CM, Wagner T, Rigonatti SP, Marcolin MA, Pascual-Leone A (2005) A sham stimulation-controlled trial of rTMS of the unaffected hemisphere in stroke patients. Neurology 64:1802–1804
113. Takeuchi N, Tada T, Toshima M, Chuma T, Matsuo Y, Ikoma K (2008) Inhibition of the unaffected motor cortex by 1 Hz repetitive transcranical magnetic stimulation enhances motor performance and training effect of the paretic hand in patients with chronic stroke. J Rehabil Med 40:298–303
114. Fregni F, Boggio PS, Valle AC, Rocha RR, Duarte J, Ferreira MJ, Wagner T, Fecteau S, Rigonatti SP, Riberto M, Freedman SD, Pascual-Leone A (2006) A sham-controlled trial of a 5-day course of repetitive transcranial magnetic stimulation of the unaffected hemisphere in stroke patients. Stroke 37:2115–2122
115. Khedr EM, Ahmed MA, Fathy N, Rothwell JC (2005) Therapeutic trial of repetitive transcranial magnetic stimulation after acute ischemic stroke. Neurology 65:466–468
116. Kim YH, You SH, Ko MH, Park JW, Lee KH, Jang SH, Yoo WK, Hallett M (2006) Repetitive transcranial magnetic stimulation-induced corticomotor excitability and associated motor skill acquisition in chronic stroke. Stroke 37:1471–1476
117. Pfurtscheller G, Klimesch W (1992) Functional topography during a visuoverbal judgment task studied with event-related desynchronization mapping. J Clin Neurophysiol 9:120–131
118. Diwakar M, Huang MX, Srinivasan R, Harrington DL, Robb A, Angeles A, Muzzatti L, Pakdaman R, Song T, Theilmann RJ, Lee RR (2011) Dual-core beamformer for obtaining highly correlated neuronal networks in MEG. Neuroimage 54:253–263

Brain–Machine Interfaces for Persons with Disabilities

Kenji Kansaku

Abstract The brain–machine interface (BMI) or brain–computer interface (BCI) is a new interface technology that utilizes neurophysiological signals from the brain to control external machines or computers. We used electroencephalography signals in a BMI system that enables environmental control and communication using the P300 paradigm, which presents a selection of icons arranged in a matrix. The subject focuses attention on one of the flickering icons in the matrix as a target. We also prepared a green/blue flicker matrix because this color combination is considered the safest chromatic combination for patients with photosensitive epilepsy. We showed that the green/blue flicker matrix was associated with a better subjective feeling of comfort than was the white/gray flicker matrix, and we also found that the green/blue flicker matrix was associated with better performance. We further added augmented reality (AR) to make an AR-BMI system, in which the user's brain signals controlled an agent robot and operated devices in the robot's environment. Thus, the user's thoughts became reality through the robot's eyes, enabling the augmentation of real environments outside of the human body. Studies along these lines may provide useful information to expand the range of activities in persons with disabilities.

Introduction

The brain–machine interface (BMI) or brain–computer interface (BCI) is a new interface technology that utilizes neurophysiological signals from the brain to control external machines or computers [1, 2]. One research approach to BMI utilizes neurophysiological signals directly from neurons or the cortical surface.

K. Kansaku (✉)
Systems Neuroscience Section, Department of Rehabilitation for Brain Functions,
Research Institute of National Rehabilitation Center for Persons with Disabilities (NRCD),
4-1 Namiki, Tokorozawa, Saitama 359-8555, Japan
e-mail: kansaku-kenji@rehab.go.jp

K. Kansaku and L.G. Cohen (eds.), *Systems Neuroscience and Rehabilitation*,
DOI 10.1007/978-4-431-54008-3_2, © Springer 2011

These approaches are categorized as invasive BMI, as they require neurosurgery [3–5]. Another approach utilizes neurophysiological signals from the brain accessed without surgery, which is called non-invasive BMI. Electroencephalography (EEG), a technique for recording neurophysiological signals using electrodes placed on the scalp, constitutes the primary non-invasive methodology for studying BMI.

Electroencephalography-based non-invasive BMI does not require neurosurgery, but is thought to provide only limited information. However, Wolpaw and McFarland succeeded in achieving two-dimensional cursor control [6] using EEG signals. They applied the EEG power spectrum, using the beta-band power for vertical cursor control and the μ-band power for horizontal cursor control. Motor imagery tasks have been used in BMI research, for example, Pfurtscheller et al. used motor imagery tasks and reported event-related beta-band synchronization and μ-wave desynchronization [7–9].

Sensory evoked signals have also been utilized in EEG-based non-invasive BMI. One popular system, the P300 speller, uses elicited P300 responses to target stimuli placed among row and column flashes [10]. Recent studies have evaluated the use of systems relying on sensory evoked signals in patients with amyotrophic lateral sclerosis and other diseases [11–13].

Our research group has applied the P300 paradigm to a BMI system that enables environmental control and communication. We tested the system on both quadriplegic and able-bodied participants and showed that participants could operate the system with little training [14, 15]. We also looked for better visual stimuli to use in the system and found that the green/blue color combination is a better visual stimulus for controlling the system [16, 17]. We then added augmented reality (AR) to make an AR-BMI system [18, 19]. This chapter introduces a series of our recent studies on BMI and discusses how these new technologies can contribute to expand the range of activities of those with disabilities.

A BMI System for Environmental Control and Communication

Our research group used EEG signals to develop a BMI system that enables environmental control and communication (Fig. 1). We modified the so-called P300 speller [10], which uses the P300 paradigm and presents a selection of icons arranged in a white/gray flicker matrix. With this protocol, the participant focuses on one icon in the matrix as the target, and each row/column or single icon of the matrix is then intensified in a random sequence. The target stimuli are presented as rare stimuli (i.e., the oddball paradigm). We elicited P300 responses to the target stimuli and then extracted and classified these responses with regard to the target.

For the visual stimuli of the BMI-based environmental control system (BMI-ECS), we first prepared four panels with white/gray flicker matrices; one each for the desk light, primitive agent-robot, television control, and hiragana spelling. These consisted of 3×3, 3×3, 6×4, and 8×10 flicker matrices, respectively. We tested the system on both quadriplegic and able-bodied participants and reported that the system could be operated effortlessly [14]. Based on the experience of this

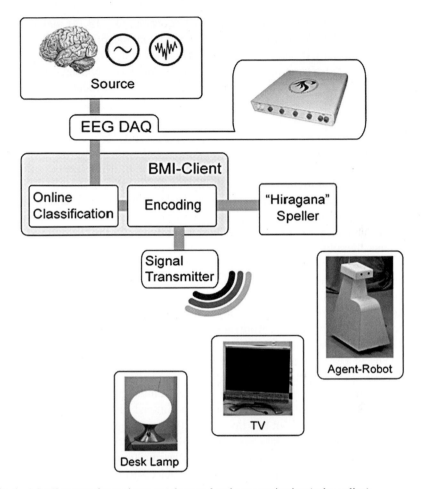

Fig. 1 A BMI system for environmental control and communication (color online)

successful preliminary experiment, we began a series of studies to build a practical BMI system for environmental control and communication, which could be useful for individuals with disabilities.

Effects of Color Combinations

Subjective Feeling of Comfort

The P300 speller has used mainly white/gray flicker matrices as visual stimuli [20–22]. It is possible that such flickering visual stimuli could induce discomfort. Parra et al. evaluated the safety of chromatic combinations in patients with photosensitive epilepsy [23]. They used five single-color stimuli (white, blue, red, yellow, and green) and four alternating-color stimuli (blue/red, red/green, green/blue, and blue/yellow with equal luminance) at four frequencies (10, 15, 20, and 30 Hz) as the visual stimuli. Under the white stimulation condition, flickering stimuli at higher frequencies, especially those greater than 20 Hz, were found to be potentially provocative. Under the alternating-color stimulation condition, as suggested by the Pokémon incidence, the 15-Hz blue/red flicker was most provocative. The green/blue chromatic flicker emerged as the safest and evoked the lowest rates of EEG spikes. Following the study of Parra et al., we conducted studies that applied a green/blue chromatic combination to elicit visually evoked responses.

In the first study, we prepared panels with 3×3 and 8×10 matrices, which were intensified using two color combinations (green/blue or white/gray), and these were used for the desk-light control and hiragana spelling. We compared the green/blue and white/gray flicker conditions, and the order of the experimental conditions (type of flicker matrix) was randomized among subjects. The flicker consisted of 100 ms of intensification and 75 ms of rest in both conditions (Fig. 2). After the experiments, the subjects were required to evaluate the conditions by their subjective feeling of comfort using a visual analogue scale. Eight non-trained able-bodied subjects (age 25–47 years; four females; all right-handed) were recruited.

This series of studies was approved by the institutional review board, and all subjects provided informed consent according to institutional guidelines. The data recordings and analyses that we applied were rather conventional. We recorded eight-channels (Fz, Cz Pz, P3, P4, Oz, PO7, and PO8 of the extended international 10–20 system) of EEG data using a cap (Guger Technologies OEG, Graz, Austria) [24, 25]. All channels were referenced to the Fpz, and grounded to the AFz. The EEG was band-pass filtered at 0.1–50 Hz, amplified with a g.Usbamp (Guger Technologies), digitized at a rate of 256 Hz, and stored. For the analyses, recorded and filtered EEG data were down-sampled to about 21 Hz. Data from 800 ms of the EEG were segmented according to the timing of the intensification. Data from the initial 100 ms were used for baseline correction. Data from the final 700 ms were used for classification purposes, using Fisher's linear discriminant analysis. First, we asked the subjects to input six letters to gather data to derive the feature vectors for the subsequent test session. The EEG data were sorted using the information on flash timing, and Fisher's linear discriminant analysis was then performed to generate the feature vector to discriminate between target and non-target. Feature vectors were derived for each condition. In the test session, visually evoked responses from EEG features were evaluated by the feature vectors. The result of the classification was construed as the maximum of the summed scores.

In the first study, the measured subjective feelings of comfort for the white/gray and green/blue flicker matrices were 55.0 and 89.0%, respectively, for the desk-light control and 38.7 and 65.1% for the hiragana spelling. The differences under each condition were significant ($p < 0.05$). We also evaluated online performance. In this experiment, each command was selected in a series of ten sequences. In addition to the observation that the green/blue flicker matrix was associated with a better subjective feeling of comfort than was the white/gray flicker matrix, the accuracy rates for the white/gray and green/blue flicker matrices were 55.8 and 80.8%, respectively, for the desk-light control and 50.8 and 75.0% for the hiragana spelling (n=8, Fig. 3) [16]. The differences under each condition were significant (p<0.05).

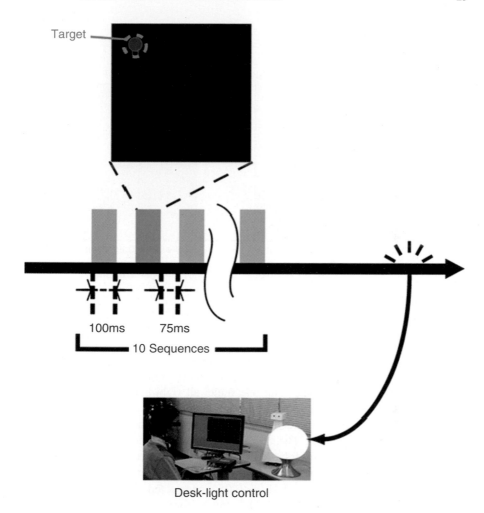

Fig. 2 Task timing

Effects of Luminance and Chromatics

Because the green/blue flicker matrix was associated with not only better subjective feelings of comfort but also better performance, we further evaluated the effects of luminance and chromatics on the visual stimulus combinations. In the second study, we prepared an 8×10 hiragana matrix for the P300 speller. Three intensification/rest flicker combinations were prepared: a white (20 cd/cm)/gray (6.5 cd/cm) flicker (L condition) matrix for the luminance flicker, a green (9.5 cd/cm)/blue (9.5 cd/cm) isoluminance flicker (C condition) matrix for the chromatic flicker, and a green (20 cd/cm)/blue (6.5 cd/cm) luminance flicker (LC condition) matrix for the luminance and chromatic flicker. The flicker consisted of 100 ms of intensification and 75 ms of rest. Luminance was measured using a chromatic meter (CS-200, Konica Minolta

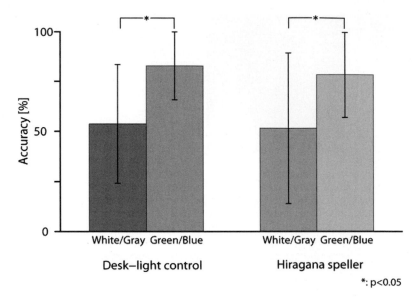

Fig. 3 Operation accuracy for the desk-light control and the hiragana speller (color online)

Sensing, Osaka, Japan). The order of the experimental conditions (type of flicker matrix) was randomized among subjects. Ten healthy, non-trained naive subjects (aged 25–47 years; nine females and one male; all right-handed) who had never participated in this study were recruited as participants.

Online performance was evaluated. In this experiment, each letter was selected in a series of ten sequences. The accuracy rate was in the order LC: 80.6% > C: 73.3% ≥ L: 71.3%. The transfer bit rates (bit/min) [26] were in the order LC: 8.14 > C: 7.03 ≥ L: 6.75. The difference in the accuracy rate between the LC and L conditions was significant ($t(9) = 2.41$, $p < 0.05$, uncorrected) (n = 10, Fig. 4) [17].

The LC condition was associated with better performance, whereas the isoluminance C condition gave similar results to the L condition. An examination of the online performance of each subject showed that one, four, and five of the ten subjects performed most accurately in the L, C, and LC conditions, respectively. This information may be used to select the best visual stimuli for situations in which the BMI system is actually used.

AR-BMI

A System Operated with a See-Through Head Mount Display

As an extension of the BMI-ECS, we combined AR with BMI. AR is a technique for live viewing of a physical real-world environment whose elements are augmented by virtual computer-generated imagery. We developed the AR-BMI because the new system can provide suitable panels to the users when they come to the area close to

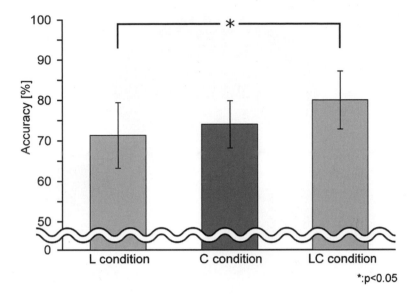

Fig. 4 The LC condition, which used the green/blue flicker matrix, was associated with better performance (color online)

the controllable devices. In this study, a USB camera was mounted on a camera platform or see-through HMD, and when the camera detects an AR marker, the pre-assigned infrared appliance becomes controllable. The AR marker's position and posture were calculated from the images detected by the camera, and a control panel for appliances was created by the AR system and superimposed on the sight of the subject's environment. When the camera detects the AR marker of the TV or desk light, a flicker panel to control it is displayed on the screen devices (Fig. 5). The AR-BMI system uses ARToolKit [27]. The subjects were required to use their brain signals to operate targets on an LCD monitor or a see-through HMD.

Two control panels of the TV and desk light were used. The TV control panel had 11 icons (power on, seven TV programs, video input, volume up and down), and the light control panel had four icons (turn on, turn off, light up, dim). We prepared the green/blue flicker matrices [17], and the duration of the intensification/rest was 100/50 ms. All icons flickered in a random order and it made a sequence. One classification was conducted per 15 sequences. Participants were required to send five commands to control both the TV and the light. Fifteen able-bodied subjects who had not previously participated in this study were recruited (aged 19–46 years; 3 females and 12 males; all right-handed).

Online performance was evaluated, and the mean accuracy rate for the TV control was 88% in the LCD monitor condition and 82.7% in the HMD condition, and these were not significantly different. In offline evaluation, these were significantly different (two-way repeated ANOVA $F_{(1,420)} = 13.6$, $p < 0.05$, Tukey–Kramer test $p < 0.05$).

The mean accuracy rate for the light control was 84% in the LCD monitor condition and 76% in the HMD condition, and these were not significantly different. These were also not significantly different in the offline evaluation (Fig. 6) [19].

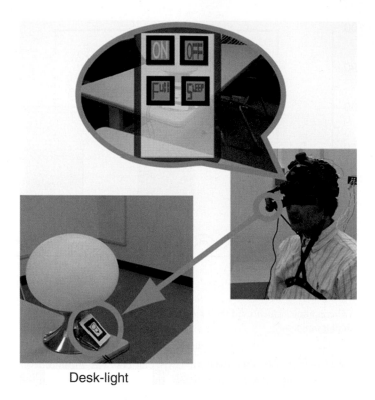

Desk-light

Fig. 5 An AR-BMI system operated with a see-through head mount display

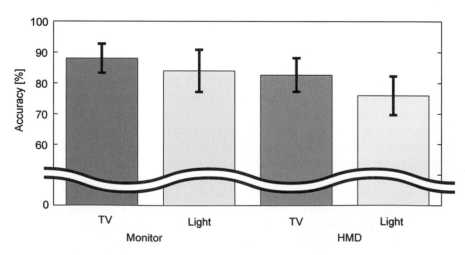

Fig. 6 Operation accuracy for the AR-BMI system with a monitor and a see-through HMD (color online)

The AR-BMI system can be operated not only by using the LCD monitor but also by using the HMD.

A System Operated Through an Agent Robot's Eye

We further prepared an agent robot for the AR-BMI system, because the new system can provide suitable panels to the users when the agent robot comes to the area close to the controllable devices, even without the appearance of the real users. In the system, when the robot's eyes detect an AR marker, the pre-assigned infrared appliance becomes controllable. The position and orientation of the AR marker were calculated from the images detected by the camera, and a control panel for the appliance was created by the AR system and superimposed on the scene detected by the robot's eyes (Fig. 7). To control our system using brain signals, we modified a Donchin P300 speller. The AR-BMI system can control both the agent robot and the desk light. The robot control panel has four icons (forward, backward, right, and left), as does the light control panel (turn on, turn off, make brighter, and make dimmer). We prepared green/blue flicker icons [17], and the duration of the intensification/rest of the flicker was 100/50 ms. All of the icons flickered in random order, which formed a sequence (600 ms). One classification was conducted every 15 sequences. Subjects were

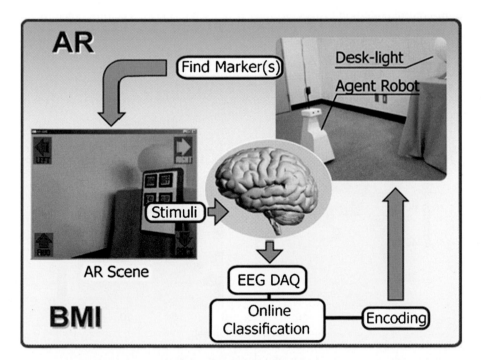

Fig. 7 An AR-BMI system operated through an agent robot's eye

required to send 15 command infrared signals to control both the robot and light. Before the trials, we checked the commands that the subjects were going to send, and then the information was used to evaluate the subjects' online performance. We also performed an offline evaluation using the recorded data.

Ten healthy, non-trained naive subjects (aged 19–39 years; two females and eight males) were recruited as participants. Using the EEG-based BMI system, the participants were first required to make the robot move to a desk light in the robot's environment. To control the robot, each command was selected in a series of 15 sequences, and the participants were required to send 15 commands. Online performance was evaluated, and the mean accuracy for controlling the robot was 90.0%.

When the robot' eyes detected the AR marker of the desk light, a flicker panel for controlling the appliance was displayed on the screen. Then, the participants had to use their brain signals to operate the light in the robot's environment through the robot's eyes. To operate the light, each command was selected in a series of 15 sequences, and the participants were required to send 15 commands. Online performance was evaluated, and the mean accuracy for light control was 80.7%.

Figure 8 shows the offline evaluation of the participant's performance under the robot-control and light-control conditions. The performance for controlling the robot and desk light differed significantly, and an interaction effect was observed by a two-way repeated ANOVA ($F_{(1,280)} = 6.53$, $p < 0.05$). *Post-hoc* testing revealed significant differences between the robot-control condition and the light-control condition (Tukey–Kramer test, $p < 0.05$) [18]. The difference might be related to the differences in the relative locations of the flicker icons on the screen [28].

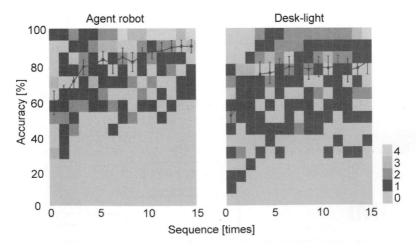

Fig. 8 Operation accuracy for the AR-BMI system (color online)

Discussion

In our series of studies, we used EEG signals for a BMI system that enables environmental control and communication using a modified P300 speller [10]. In a preliminary experiment, we prepared four panels with white/gray flicker matrices, one each for the desk light, primitive agent-robot, television control, and hiragana spelling. We tested them on both quadriplegic and able-bodied participants and found that both groups succeeded in operating the system without much training [14]. We then prepared a green/blue flicker matrix for the visual stimuli, because this color combination is considered to be the safest [23]. As expected, we found that the green/blue flicker matrix was associated with a better subjective feeling of comfort than was the white/gray flicker matrix. Further, we found that the green/blue flicker matrix was associated with better performance than was the white/gray flicker matrix [16, 17].

To increase accuracy when operating the BMI system and to develop better classification methods [12, 20, 29, 30], some studies have attempted to identify better, more-efficient experimental settings by manipulating factors such as matrix size and duration of intensification [21], channel set of the EEG [22], and flash pattern of the flicker matrix [31]. We proposed a method that combines luminance and chromatic information to increase the accuracy of performance using the P300 BMI, and this method can be applied with the methods proposed in the aforementioned reports.

Our BMI system equipped with the P300 paradigm was tested on both patients with quadriplegia and able-bodied persons, and it worked well for environmental control and communication [14, 15]. Note that the participants could use the system with little training. The participants only had to input six letters to gather data to derive the feature vectors for the subsequent test session, and this took only a few minutes. Using adequate visual stimuli, such as the green/blue flicker matrix, also helped to improve the system. Note that directed attention is needed to elicit P300-related responses, and this is not necessarily the direction of eye-gaze; therefore, this system may potentially benefit persons who cannot move their eyes freely.

One specific merit of the P300 speller algorithms is that we can easily translate the subject's thoughts as a command pre-assigned to each icon. Therefore, our system can be used for various applications in environmental control and communication. This should also help to expand the range of options for applications. For example, it was possible to combine AR techniques with BMI to make an AR-BMI system [18, 19]. The new AR-BMI system provided suitable panels to the users when they or their agent came to an area close to the controllable devices. Further, in our recent study, in which we used a hybrid BMI platform (a combined platform with a P300-based BMI and a sensorimotor rhythm-based BMI) [32], we prepared life-sized robot arms that could supply driving forces to a wearer's upper-limb motions, such as reaching and grasping, and developed an assist suit for persons with physical disabilities and those undergoing occupational therapy (Fig. 9) [33].

To deliver the new technologies to persons with disabilities, we made an in-house BMI system for environmental control and communication [32]. The hardware system includes an EEG amp, electrodes, cap, PC, programmable IR remote

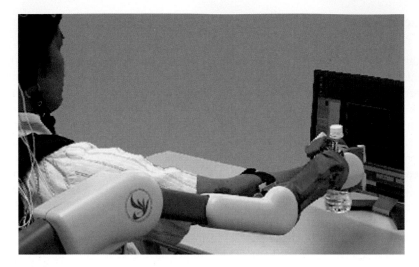

Fig. 9 A BMI-based assist-suite for the upper limb

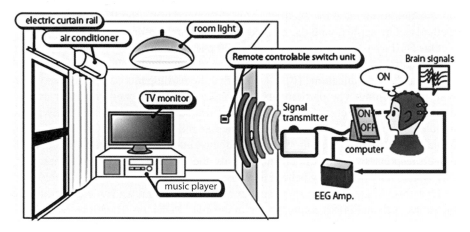

Fig. 10 A diagram of a BMI-based intelligent house (color online)

controller, and interfaces for home electronics. The software system has functions for EEG acquisition, analysis, classification, stimulus presentation, application control (writing, e-mail, home electronics control, etc.). One EEG amp has four data channels and can be connected to other EEG amps to increase the number of data channels. This EEG amp also has two external input channels. The EEG amp and PC are easy to handle and transport. We started clinical experiments for patients with paralysis using the in-house set.

For practical applications of the new BMI technologies, ethical issues must also be considered, although the system using the P300 speller algorithms may be safer than other BMI technologies because it simply elicits implemented brain responses and does not require constructing new circuits in the brain with extensive training. Our experience developing BMI technology has suggested that it is useful for supporting those with disabilities, and one future direction of study would be to build BMI-based intelligent houses (Fig. 10).

Conclusion

We used electroencephalography signals in a BMI system that enables environmental control and communication using the P300 paradigm, which presents a selection of icons arranged in a matrix. We showed that the green/blue flicker matrix was associated with a better subjective feeling of comfort than was the white/gray flicker matrix, and we also found that the green/blue flicker matrix was associated with better performance. We further added AR to make an AR-BMI system, in which the user's brain signals controlled an agent robot and operated devices in the robot's environment. BMI technology could be used to build BMI-based intelligent houses to support those with disabilities.

Acknowledgements These studies were conducted with the NRCD post-doctoral fellows Drs. Kouji Takano, Tomoaki Komatsu, Shiro Ikegami, and Naoki Hata. I thank Dr. Günter Edlinger for his help, and Drs. Yasoichi Nakajima and Motoi Suwa for their continuous encouragement.

References

1. Lebedev MA, Nicolelis MA (2006) Brain–machine interfaces: past, present and future. Trends Neurosci 29:536–546
2. Birbaumer N, Cohen LG (2007) Brain–computer interfaces: communication and restoration of movement in paralysis. J Physiol 579:621–636
3. Hochberg L, Serruya M, Friehs G, Mukand J, Saleh M, Caplan AH, Branner A, Chen D, Penn R, Donoghue J (2006) Neuronal ensemble control of prosthetic devices by a human with tetraplegia. Nature 442:164–171
4. Jarosiewicz B, Chase SM, Fraser GW, Velliste M, Kass RE, Schwartz AB (2008) Functional network reorganization during learning in a brain–computer interface paradigm. Proc Natl Acad Sci USA 105:19486–19491
5. Miller KJ, Schalk G, Fetz EE, den Nijs M, Ojemann JG, Rao RP (2010) Cortical activity during motor execution, motor imagery, and imagery-based online feedback. Proc Natl Acad Sci USA 107:4430–4435
6. Wolpaw JR, McFarland DJ (2004) Control of a two-dimensional movement signal by a noninvasive brain–computer interface in humans. Proc Natl Acad Sci USA 101:17849–17854
7. Guger C, Edlinger G, Harkam W, Niedermayer I, Pfurtscheller G (2003) How many people are able to operate an EEG-based brain–computer interface (BCI)? IEEE Trans Neural Syst Rehabil Eng 11:145–147
8. Bai O, Mari Z, Vorbach S, Hallett M (2005) Asymmetric spatiotemporal patterns of event-related desynchronization preceding voluntary sequential finger movements: a high-resolution EEG study. Clin Neurophysiol 116:1213–1221
9. Pfurtscheller G, Brunner C, Schlogl A, Lopes da Silva FH (2006) Mu rhythm (de)synchronization and EEG single-trial classification of different motor imagery tasks. NeuroImage 31:153–159

10. Farwell LA, Donchin E (1988) Talking off the top of your head: toward a mental prosthesis utilizing event-related brain potentials. Electroencephalogr Clin Neurophysiol 70:510–523
11. Piccione F, Giorgi F, Tonin P, Priftis K, Giove S, Silvoni S, Palmas G, Beverina F (2006) P300-based brain computer interface: reliability and performance in healthy and paralysed participants. Clin Neurophysiol 117:531–537
12. Sellers EW, Donchin E (2006) A P300-based brain–computer interface: initial tests by ALS patients. Clin Neurophysiol 117:538–548
13. Nijboer F, Sellers EW, Mellinger J, Jordan MA, Matuz T, Furdea A, Halder S, Mochty U, Krusienski DJ, Vaughan TM, Wolpaw JR, Birbaumer N, Kubler A (2008) A P300-based brain–computer interface for people with amyotrophic lateral sclerosis. Clin Neurophysiol 119:1909–1916
14. Komatsu T, Hata N, Nakajima Y, Kansaku K (2008) A non-training EEG-based BMI system for environmental control. Neurosci Res Suppl 61:S251
15. Ikegami S, Takano K, Komatsu T, Saeki N, Kansaku K (2009) Operation of a BMI based environmental control system by patients with cervical spinal cord injury. Neuroscience meeting planner. Society for Neuroscience, Chicago. Online Program No. 664.16
16. Takano K, Ikegami S, Komatsu T, Kansaku K (2009) Green/blue flicker matrices for the P300 BCI improve the subjective feeling of comfort. Neurosci Res Suppl 65:S182
17. Takano K, Komatsu T, Hata N, Nakajima Y, Kansaku K (2009) Visual stimuli for the P300 brain–computer interface: a comparison of white/gray and green/blue flicker matrices. Clin Neurophysiol 120:1562–1566
18. Kansaku K, Hata N, Takano K (2010) My thoughts through a robot's eyes: an augmented reality–brain machine interface. Neurosci Res 66:219–222
19. Takano K, Hata N, Nakajima Y, Kansaku K (2010) AR-BMI operated with a HMD: effects of channel selection. Neuroscience meeting planner. Society for Neuroscience, San Diego. Online Program No. 295.18
20. Kaper M, Meinicke P, Grossekathoefer U, Lingner T, Ritter H (2004) BCI Competition 2003–Data set IIb: support vector machines for the P300 speller paradigm. IEEE Trans Biomed Eng 51:1073–1076
21. Sellers EW, Krusienski DJ, McFarland DJ, Vaughan TM, Wolpaw JR (2006) A P300 event-related potential brain–computer interface (BCI): the effects of matrix size and inter stimulus interval on performance. Biol Psychol 73:242–252
22. Krusienski DJ, Sellers EW, McFarland DJ, Vaughan TM, Wolpaw JR (2008) Toward enhanced P300 speller performance. J Neurosci Methods 167:15–21
23. Parra J, Lopes da Silva FH, Stroink H, Kalitzin S (2007) Is colour modulation an independent factor in human visual photosensitivity? Brain 130:1679–1689
24. Krusienski DJ, Sellers EW, Vaughan TM (2007) Common spatio-temporal patterns for the p300 speller. In: 3rd International IEEE EMBS conference on neural engineering, Kohala Coast, Hawaii, USA, pp 421–424
25. Lu S, Guan C, Zhang H (2008) Unsupervised brain computer interface based on inter-subject information. In: 30th Annual international IEEE EMBS conference, Vancouver, British Columbia, Canada, pp 638–641
26. Wolpaw JR, Birbaumer N, McFarland DJ, Pfurtscheller G, Vaughan TM (2002) Brain–computer interfaces for communication and control. Clin Neurophysiol 113:767–791
27. Kato H, Billinghurst M (1999) Marker tracking and HMD calibration for a video-based augmented reality conferencing system. In: International workshop on augmented reality, San Francisco, USA, pp 85–94
28. Cheng M, Gao X, Gao S, Xu D (2002) Design and implementation of a brain–computer interface with high transfer rates. IEEE Trans Biomed Eng 49:1181–1186
29. Donchin E, Spencer KM, Wijesinghe R (2000) The mental prosthesis: assessing the speed of a P300-based brain–computer interface. IEEE Trans Rehabil Eng 8:174–179
30. Bostanov V (2004) BCI Competition 2003 – data sets Ib and IIb: feature extraction from event-related brain potentials with the continuous wavelet transform and the t-value scalogram. IEEE Trans Biomed Eng 51:1057–1061

31. Townsend G, LaPallo BK, Boulay CB, Krusienski DJ, Frye GE, Hauser CK, Schwartz NE, Vaughan TM, Wolpaw JR, Sellers EW (2010) A novel P300-based brain–computer interface stimulus presentation paradigm: moving beyond rows and columns. Clin Neurophysiol 121:1109–1120
32. Komatsu T, Takano K, Nakajima Y, Kansaku K (2009) A BMI based environmental control system: a combination of sensorimotor rhythm, P300, and virtual reality. Neuroscience meeting planner. Society for Neuroscience, Chicago. Online Program No. 360.14
33. Komatsu T, Takano K, Ikegami S, Kansaku K (2010) A development of a BCI-based OT-assist suit for paralyzed upper extremities. Neuroscience meeting planner. Society for Neuroscience, San Diego. Online Program No. 295.9

Brain–Machine Interfaces Based on Computational Model

Yasuharu Koike, Hiroyuki Kambara, Natsue Yoshimura, and Duk Shin

Abstract The research about brain computer interface or brain machine interface has been widely developed in this decade. Implant methods are already used for eye or ear as retinal implant or cochlear implant, these devices stimulate peripheral nerve. In this case, the stimulus site is peripheral and the information from each sensor is input signal of the brain. Brain Machine Interface measure or stimulate neuron in the brain directly and decode neuronal firings to generate information. It is impossible to measure all neuron activities from brain, because of enormous quantity of neurons and also the function is unknown. So anatomical knowledge, such as a cortical homunculus of the primary motor cortex and the primary somatosensory cortex, or neural scientific knowledge is used.

The process of movement from the primary motor cortex to muscle is forward direction, and the number of neurons are decrease in this process. The generation of muscle activities are straightforward. In the field of motor control, motor command generation is still open problem. There are many theories are proposed. In order to evaluate or verify these theories, the technique of BMI is also useful. In this chapter, we introduce musculo-skeletal model and computational model for movement, and also some examples of BMI/BCI.

Y. Koike (✉)
Tokyo Institute of Technology, 4259-R2-15, Nagatsuta-cho, Midori-ku,
Yokohama, Kanagawa 226-8503, Japan
and
JST CREST, 4-1-8, Honmachi, Kawaguchi, Saitama, Japan
e-mail: koike@pi.titech.ac.jp

H. Kambara • N. Yoshimura • D. Shin
Tokyo Institute of Technology, 4259-R2-15, Nagatsuta-cho, Midori-ku,
Yokohama, Kanagawa 226-8503, Japan

K. Kansaku and L.G. Cohen (eds.), *Systems Neuroscience and Rehabilitation*,
DOI 10.1007/978-4-431-54008-3_3, © Springer 2011

Introduction

The research about brain computer interface or brain machine interface has been widely developed in this decade. brain machine interface measure or stimulate neuron in the brain directly and decode neuronal firings to generate information. It is impossible to measure all neuron activities from brain, because of enormous quantity of neurons and also it is difficult to decode the brain signals, because the function is complicated and still unknown. So anatomical knowledge or scientific knowledge, such as a cortical homunculus of the primary motor cortex and the primary somatosensory cortex, the neural representation of the primary motor cortex are used. These area are related the movement and sense of touch. In the field of motor control, motor command generation is still open problem. There are many theories are proposed.

Since 1999, when Chapin et al. [1] controlled arm movement of a robot in one degree of freedom from the neural activity of the motor cortex of a rat, much development and research has been done in this field. Carmena et al. [2] succeeded in reconstructing arm movement of a robot in three degrees of freedom and grip force from the neural activity of the premotor cortex, primary motor cortex and posterior parietal cortical area of a monkey. In addition, Musallam et al. [3] extracted high level signals, such as the goal of a movement, the preference and motivation of a subject from the neuron signal of the parietal reach region (PRR) and area 5 which are the major pathways of visually guided movement. Recently, Hochberg et al. [4] succeeded in controlling a computer cursor on a two dimensional display from the signal of the primary motor cortex of the brain of an actual human.

In order to implement a brain machine interface system similar to a human arm, reconstructing the position and force information of the arm from the neural activity of the brain is necessary. For example, if we consider when a human picks up an object, the human moves his arm to the object position from the original position, then gives proper force depending on the weight of the object. Like this the reconstruction of the force information is an important factor in the implementation of brain machine interface system. We used EMG signals to reconstruct the position and force information, simultaneously. EMG signals reflect muscle tensions, so, we can reconstruct arm posture, joint torque and stiffness from the EMG signals, precisely.

Until now, several hypotheses have been proposed to find out the relationship between the neural activities of the primary motor cortex and motor control. Among these hypotheses, there are hypothesis that the neural activities of the primary motor cortex encode movement direction [5], a hypothesis that the neural activities encode force [6], and a hypothesis that the neural activities encode both of movement direction and force [7]. Nevertheless these endeavors, we have yet known the exact relationship between the neuron activities in M1 and motor control.

In order to evaluate or verify these theories, the technique of BMI is also useful.

Brain Machine Interface

One of the most important things is where we measure the brain signals for the brain machine interface (Fig. 1). The topological mapping of the brain is well known and the properties of the neuron activities have been analyzing from the view points of the correlation with the behavior. From these results, the useful information, such as the movement direction, muscle activities, joint torque and so on, is extracted from the brain signals, and this is called a decoder.

Another important thing is that how does the brain control our body. This is included that what is motor command, what is control law, and so on. Because the information representation is tied to the algorithm of control. For example, the neuron activities of primary motor cortex would be related muscle activities. Because the primary motor cortex is one of the output of the brain to the muscles, and the representation of those neurons are coupled with peripheral sensors or actuators. A desired trajectories or a target of the movement would be represent in the brain before the movement is executed, and the current state of the body would be fed back to the brain and compared with the desired trajectories to compensate the error.

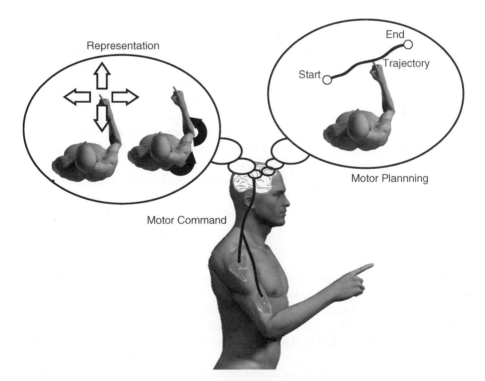

Fig. 1 Where do we measure brain activities? The primary motor cortex is one of the major places. Because the motor command is send to the muscles. The neuron activities are related to the movement direction, joint angle, joint torque and so on. In the frontal cortex, the intention, target place, or planed trajectory may be represented (color online)

However, it is thought that not only one region but also the multiple regions are related to the higher information such as an intention of the execution or the environmental recognition. It is likely to be represent the different way from the peripheral information. Furthermore, if it is hard to know "when" those information is handled, it would be difficult to decode the information or encode them in appropriate timing.

Computational neuroscience will support the direction of the analysis. Some assumption of the model or the computer simulation will help the understanding of the decoding or encoding of the neural information.

In this chapter, BMI based on musculo-skeletal model will be introduced and the computational model will be introduced.

BMI Based on Musculo-Skeletal Model

The aim of the our study is to computationally reconstruct movements from brain activities and to use them as a basis for a new BMI system. We recorded movement-related neural activity of the primary motor cortex (M1) as well as Electromyographic (EMG) activity in a Japanese monkey as it performed an arm-reaching task. We attempted to estimate the movement trajectories from the combination of the neuronal and the physiological muscle data.

In our previous research studies, we computed not only the motion and joint torque of the arm, but also the equilibrium position and joint stiffness from the EMG signals [8–10]. These results indicate that the EMG signals reflect the muscle tension and are correlated with the movements. From the anatomical viewpoint, the primary motor cortex M1 controls the tractus corticospinalis and the subcortical motor areas, resulting in fine and smooth movements of the dedicated muscles. Thus, muscle activities are useful to estimate them. The muscle force was produced in accordance with the motor commands. Shoulder and elbow joint angles were then estimated from the muscle activity. The arm trajectory was calculated from the time series of the joint angles.

Mykin Muscle Model

Earlier arm models have been proposed using two kinematic degrees of freedom in the horizontal plane [11–16]. Based on these studies, we suggested the Mykin model, in which the human arm in the horizontal plane was modeled as a two-link manipulator with six monoarticular muscles and two biarticular muscles.

In Fig. 2, the mechanical action of the bicep is shown as a rack-and-pinion gear and a spring connected in series [17]. Here, we used the Kelvin–Voigt model, consisting of an elastic element for static isometric contraction [18]. Muscle tension T could be determined from muscle stiffness $k(u)$ and the stretch length of a muscle $\{l_r(u) - l(\theta)\}$ as follows:

$$T = k(u)\{l_r(u) - l(\theta)\} \tag{1}$$

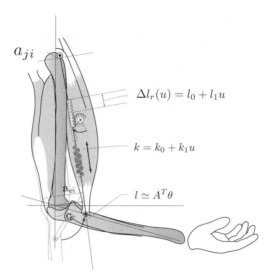

$$\Delta l_r(u) = l_0 + l_1 u$$

$$k = k_0 + k_1 u$$

$$l \simeq A^T \theta$$

Fig. 2 Mykin model and changes in limb position. The mechanical action of the elbow flexor muscle (biceps) is shown as a rack-and-pinion gear and a spring. When the muscle activation increased, the pinion rotated, and the rack pulled on the spring. Muscle length changes as a result of muscle activations and changes of the joint angles. For isometric contraction, muscle tension T can be written as a quadratic function of muscle activation and joint angle. Muscle length changes as a result of muscle activation ($\Delta l_r(u)$) and changes the joint angle (l)

$$
\begin{aligned}
k(u) &= k_0 + k_1 u \\
l_r(u) &= L_{bias} - \Delta L_{eq} \\
&= L_{bias} - \{L_{eq}(0) - L_{eq}(u)\} \\
&= L^*_{bias} - L_{eq}(u) \\
l(\theta) &= L(0) - L(\theta) \simeq A^T \theta
\end{aligned}
\tag{2}
$$

Here, the parameters k_0 and k_1 in the muscle stiffness $k(u)$ are the intrinsic elasticity and the elasticity, respectively. The muscle stiffness $k(u)$ is represented by linear functions of muscle activation u [13, 15, 19]. For muscles, the two different change of muscle length could be distinguished. First, $l_r(u)$ denotes the deviation of equilibrium length. We assumed that $l_r(u)$ could be contracted by only the muscle activation u. L_{bias} represents a bias term and ΔL_{eq} is the deviation of equilibrium length between the equilibrium length $L_{eq}(0)$ when u is zero and the current equilibrium length $L_{eq}(u)$. L^*_{bias} denotes a bias term that is set so that $l_r(u) - l(0)$ is not negative. The parameter l_0 is the intrinsic rest length when u is zero, and l_1 is a constant.

Second, $l(\theta)$ denotes the current muscle length with the current joint angle θ. $L(0)$ denotes the muscle length when the joint angle is 0, $L(\theta)$ denotes the current muscle length at the current joint angle. It could be simplified as arc ($A^T \theta$). Consequently, (3) expressed each muscles tension T_i as a quadratic function of the muscle activation u,

$$T_i(u,\theta) = (k_0^i + k_1^i u_i)\left(l_0^i + l_1^i u_i - \sum_j a_{ji}\theta_j \right), \tag{3}$$

where $a_{ji} > 0$ $(i = 1,2,\cdots,8; j = s,e)$ is the length of the moment arm. Each moment arm A_n for different postures was denoted as shown in (4).

$$A_n = \begin{pmatrix} a_{11} & \cdots & a_{1i} \\ \cdots\cdots\cdots\cdots \\ a_{j1} & \cdots & a_{ji} \end{pmatrix} \tag{4}$$

Joint torque τ_j could be determined using muscle i acting on joint j:

$$\tau_j(u,\theta) = \sum_i A_n T_i(u_i,\theta) \tag{5}$$

Joint stiffness is defined by the following differential operator:

$$R_{jk}(u,\theta) = -\frac{\partial \tau_j}{\partial \theta_k} = -\frac{\partial \left(\sum_i A_n T_i(u_i,\theta) \right)}{\partial \theta_k} \tag{6}$$

Assuming that muscle activation u_i is proportional to the EMG level, we could estimate stiffness directly by using (6). From the estimated joint stiffness R_{jk}, the hand stiffness K can be obtained using the following equation:

$$K = (J^T)^{-1} R_{jk} J^{-1} \tag{7}$$

Here, J denotes the Jacobian matrix of kinematics transformation.

Muscle Activation

Several studies have investigated the relationship between surface EMG signals and muscle force [9, 20–24]. Surface EMG signals are spatiotemporally convoluted action potentials of the muscle membranes, and involve not only descending central motor commands, but also reflex motor commands generated from sensory feedback signals. The muscle activation, therefore, is presumed to contribute to an increase in joint torque and stiffness. The rectified, filtered, and normalized EMG signals were used as the muscle activation u of (1), (3), (5), and (6).

Estimation of Joint Torque and Impedance

Based on the Kelvin–Voigt model, we proposed a mathematical muscle model using a quadratic function for muscle activation. With our simple model, we were able to obtain a close estimation of joint torque for force-regulation tasks, and produce zero torque with or without co-contraction as shown in Fig. 3.

In addition, the proposed method, which uses an equation of differentiated torque, would be effective in estimating stiffness. We confirmed that our results correlated with stiffness measured by the perturbation method in various positions as shown in Fig. 4.

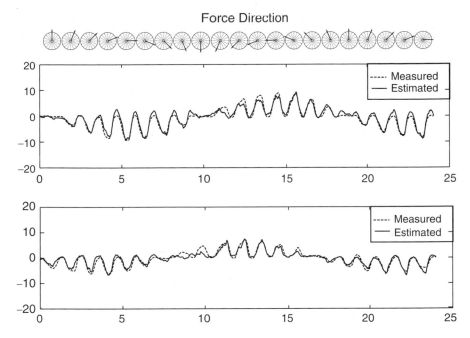

Force Direction

Fig. 3 Estimated and measured time-varying joint torque during the typical task (24 s) of Experiment I. The *arrows* in the *circles* over part A show the target directions of the force vectors on the target direction. Each raw EMG signal shows the muscle activation during force regulation task. *Dotted lines* are torque measured with a torque sensor and the *solid lines* are estimated torque using the Mykin model

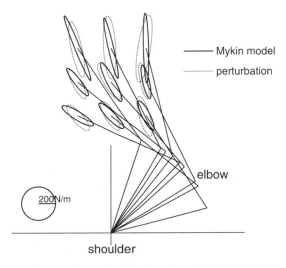

Fig. 4 Comparison of stiffness measured by the perturbation method and stiffness estimated from the Mykin model while subject was maintaining posture. *Dotted ellipses* show the estimated stiffness using Mykin model and *solid ellipses* are measurements by the perturbation method

The posture on which joint torques become zeros is the equilibrium posture. These equilibrium posture can be calculated using this kind musculo-skeletal model. As this chapter, joint properties, such as torque, stiffness, and angles, are estimated from EMG signals. If EMG activities are estimated from the neuron activities, these joint properties also estimated from only the neuron activities.

Motor Control-Learning Model

It is still open problem that how does the brain control our body. When the brain signals are decoded to the command, the representation of the information is important. For example, if the trajectory is planed in the brain before the execution, these information can be extracted from the neuron activities. If only the target is represented in the brain for execution, the trajectories would be difficult to decode from the neuron activities directly.

The computational model estimate the theoretical framework for the motor control. If only target position produce the motor command for the movement without any motor planning, the target position would be represented in the brain. And after decode the target position, the model can control the robot which has different dynamics from the human. In this chapter, our computational model is introduced.

Computational Model

Figure 5 illustrates architecture of the motor control-learning model for a reaching task. The model consists of three main modules, inverse statics model (ISM), feedback controller (FBC), and forward dynamics model (FDM). The FBC is composed of actor and critic units, which correspond to a controller and value function estimator respectively in the actor-critic method.

At the beginning of each trial, a target point of reaching is given as a desired state x^d to the model. This x^d is kept constant at the target point throughout the trial. The ISM receives x^d as an input and generates a time-invariant motor command u^{ism}. If the ISM was trained correctly, u^{ism} shifts the equilibrium of the arm to the target point. On the other hand, at time t, the FBC receives a state error between desired state x^d and future state $\hat{x}_{future}(t - \Delta t)$ predicted by the FDM Δt second before time t. The FBC, then, transforms the state error into a feedback motor command $u^{fbc}(t)$. The sum of u^{ism} and $u^{fbc}(t)$ is sent to the arm as a total motor command $u(t)$. Based on the total motor command $u(t)$ and the state $x(t)$, the FDM predicts next state $\hat{x}_{next}(t)$ and also future state $\hat{x}_{future}(t)$.

The three modules improve their performance in the following way. A teaching signal for FDM's prediction $\hat{x}_{next}(t)$ is given by observing the actual state at time $t + \Delta t$. Therefore, the FDM can be trained in normal supervised learning manner, in which the error signal is determined as:

$$E_{fdm}(t) = x(t + \Delta t) - \hat{x}_{next}(t). \tag{8}$$

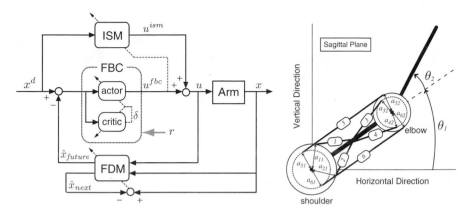

Fig. 5 The architecture of motor control-learning model: The model has three main modules, inverse statics model (ISM), feedback controller (FBC), and forward dynamics model (FDM). The FBC is composed of actor and critic units, which correspond to a controller and value function estimator respectively in the actor-critic method. The ISM generates a feed-forward motor command u^{ism} that shifts the equilibrium state of the arm to the desired state x^d. On the other hand, the FBC generates a feedback motor command u^{fbc} that reduces the error between the desired state x^d and the future state $\hat{x}_{future}$ predicted by the FDM. The error signal for the ISM is the feedback motor command u^{fbc}. Meanwhile, the teaching signal for the FDM is the state of the arm x observed at next time instant. The FBC is trained by the actor-critic method so as to maximize the cumulative reward r. The temporal difference error δ related to the reward r is used as the reinforcer and error signal for the actor and critic units, respectively

On the other hand, the ISM is trained with the feedback-error-learning scheme in which the error signal for ISM's output u^{ism} is FDM's output, that is,

$$E_{ism}(t) = u^{fbc}(t). \qquad (9)$$

Finally, the FBC is trained with the actor-critic method. The signal used to improve both actor and critic units is TD (temporal difference) error δ. The value of δ is determined from a reward signal r and state-value of the state error $(x^d - \hat{x}_{future})$ estimated by the critic unit. The TD error δ serves as an error signal for the critic unit. Meanwhile, it serves as a reinforcement signal for the actor unit.

Reaching Motions

Our model learn the equilibrium posture. Because only posture state is target. However, if we change the target posture to the end point of the movement at the initial time, our model produces the smooth movement by spring-like muscle properties. We show how reaching motion changed during the learning process. Figure 6 illustrates reaching motions simulated with sets of weight parameters just after 1,000th, 5,000th, 10,000th, and 100,000th trial. The tangential velocity profiles of

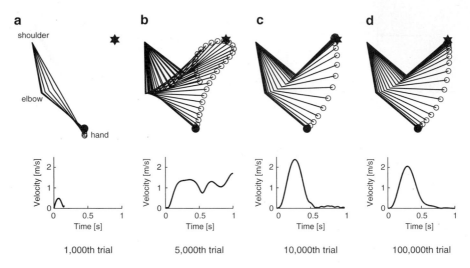

Fig. 6 Reaching motions during learning process: (**a**) 1,000th trial, (**b**) 5,000th trial, (**c**) 10,000th trial, (**d**) 100,000th trial. *Upper* and *lower plots* in each of (**a**)–(**d**) illustrate arm's motion and tangential velocity profile of the hand from time 0 to 1 s, respectively. *White circles* in the *upper plots* denote the locations of the hand during each trial. On the other hand, *black circles* and *hexagrams* denote initial positions of the hand and target positions, respectively. The joint angles at the initial and target positions in all of the trials are set as $(\theta_1(0), \theta_2(0)) = (-80, 40)$ and $(\theta_1^{trg}, \theta_2^{trg}) = (-40, 80)$, respectively

the hand are also plotted under the illustrations of the arm's motions. We set initial and target states as $\theta(0) = (-40, 80, 0, 0)$ and $\theta^{trg} = (-80, 40, 0, 0)$ for these demonstrations. At the early stage of the learning process (1,000th trial), the elbow joint was extended and the arm got away from the target (Fig. 6a). As a result, the arm got out of the work space and the reaching ended up in failure. The reaching at 5,000th trial also failed. However, considerable improvement can be seen in the behavioral output. Unlike 1,000th trial, the arm once moved toward the target as seen in Fig. 6b. Although the arm did not stop at the target, it remained within the work space. As the number of trials increases up to 10,000, the motor control-learning model became able to stop the arm at the target and hold it there as seen in Fig. 6c. Although the velocity profile is almost bell-shaped, there is a small bump around $t = 0.5$ s, indicating a lack of smooth deceleration of the arm. This small bump in the velocity profile seems to result from a small corrective motion that is seen around the target point. At the final stage of the learning process (100,000th trial), no corrective movement is observed in arm's motion and the velocity profile became smooth bell-shape typically observed in point-to-point reaching movements of adult human (Fig. 6d).

Dependence of Movement Accuracy on the Target Position

To see how accurately the motor control-learning model became able to reach the targets through training trials, we simulated reaching movements toward 900

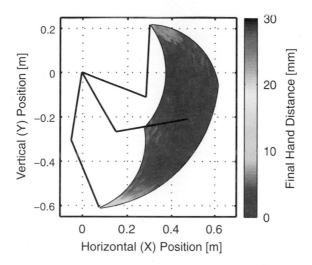

Fig. 7 Accuracy of reaching movements toward 900 targets: The *final hand distance*, the distance between target and hand position at the end of reaching movement, is displayed on the target position in the color map. The origin is set at the shoulder position and three stick figures of the arm are superimposed so as to illustrate the relative size of target area against the arm. All reaching movements are simulated using a set of weight parameters acquired with 100,000 training trials. The average and standard deviation of the 900 *final hand distances* are 3.37 mm and 1.56 mm, respectively (color online)

different targets. We used a set of weight parameters just after 100,000th trial to implement the control system. As a measure of the accuracy of reaching movement, we adopted the *final hand distance*, the distance between the target point and the hand position at the last moment of each trial. For each of the 900 targets, ten reaching movements starting from ten randomly chosen initial states were simulated. The average value of ten *final hand distances* against the same target is converted into color grade and shown on the position of corresponding target to represent the accuracy of reaching as the color map (Fig. 7). For almost all of the targets, the hand reached the points within 10 mm around the target points. The average and standard deviation of the *final hand distances* among all targets are 3.37 mm and 1.57 mm, respectively. Therefore, it can be said that our model succeeded in achieving highly accurate reaching through the successful learning process.

Comparing the Reaching Movement to the Human Movement

Figure 8 shows hand trajectories of point-to-point reaching movements executed by the subjects and those simulated by our model. Hand paths and tangential velocity profiles are shown in the figure. Gently curved hand paths were obtained both in the reaching movements of the subjects and our model. For almost all of the movements, the hand paths of the subjects and our model overlap with each other on most parts between the initial and target points. Furthermore, smooth and bell-shaped

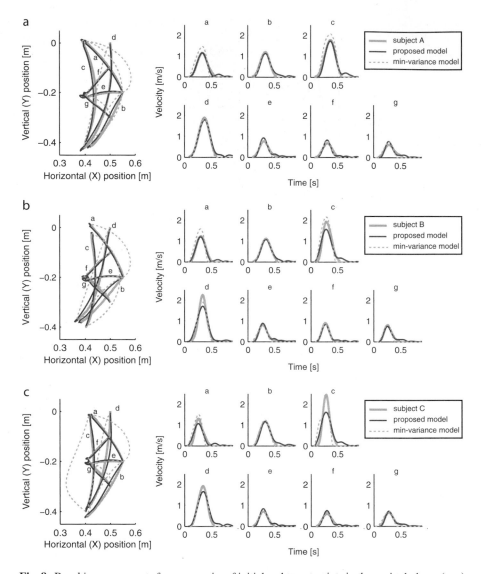

Fig. 8 Reaching movements for seven pairs of initial and target points in the sagittal plane: (**a–c**) Hand trajectory data of subject (**a–c**) (*gray solid lines*), those simulated by our model (*blue solid lines*), and those simulated by the minimum-variance model (*green dashed lines*). *Left side plots* in each of (**a–c**) illustrate hand paths of reaching movements for seven target pairs ('a', … , 'g'). *Right side plots* illustrate corresponding hand tangential velocity profiles. The velocity profiles are aligned so that the timing of peak velocity coincides with each other (color online)

curves in the velocity profiles of the subjects are reproduced well by our model. Although there are a few movements in which the peek velocities differ between the subjects and our model [movement 'c' and 'd' in (b) and (c)], the hand tangential velocity profiles in the simulation reasonably overlap with the subject's data.

BMI/BCI

Our brain machine interface is based on muscle activities. Arm movements are estimated from EMG activities which are estimated from the primary motor cortex using a three layer artificial neural network with modular architecture [25].

BMI

We trained a Japanese monkey (*Macaca fuscata*; male, 7.4 kg) to perform a continuous arm reaching task. The task, as shown in Fig. 9, consisted of pushing the buttons Hold-C-A-B, Hold-C-D-B, Hold-D-B-A, and Hold-D-C-A. First the monkey pushes the hold button for 1 s when the hold signal turns on. If the monkey succeeds in pushing the hold button for 1 s, then the C button turns on and the monkey has to push the button within 1 s. After pushing the C button, the A button turns on. As in the case of the C button, if the monkey pushes the button for 1 s, then finally the B button turns on, the monkey should push the button for 1 s. The monkey received juice rewards if the task was completely succeeded.

Estimation Result of Filtered EMG Signals from Neural Activity of Primary Motor Cortex

EMG signals were measured in nine muscles related to the four degrees of freedom (Fig. 10 and Table 1). The estimation of the filtered EMG signals is obtained by simply linearized the neural activities of the primary motor cortex with a linear regression method.

$$fEMG_i(t + \delta t) = \sum_{j=1}^{m} \omega_{ij} n_j(t) + bias \tag{10}$$

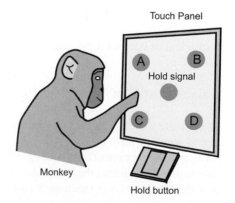

Fig. 9 Behavioral task: The monkey sat in a primate chair with its head fixing and facing a touch panel equipped with five lamps and five buttons was trained to perform a continuous arm reaching task (color online)

Fig. 10 Four degrees of
freedom arm movement

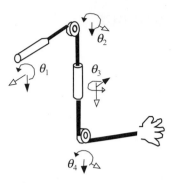

Table 1 The muscles measured EMG signals

θ_1	Adduction	Pectoralis major, teres major
	Abduction	Deltoid, deltoideus
θ_2	Extension	Deltoid, teres major, triceps brachii C.L., T. B. C. laterale
	Flexion	Deltoid, pectoralis major, biceps brachii, deltoideus
θ_3	Medial rotation	Deltoid, pectoralis major, teres major, deltoideus
	Lateral rotation	Deltoid, infraspinatus, deltoideus
θ_4	Extension	Triceps brachii caput longus, triceps brachii caput laterale
	Flexion	Biceps brachii, brachialis

Here, $fEMG_i$ and n_j describe the i th filtered EMG signal from j th neuron. δt is the delay between the neuron activity of the primary motor cortex and the EMG signals. The weighting-factor ω_{ij} represents the strength influence from neuron j on the muscle i.

We estimated the filtered EMG signals from 105 neurons in the primary motor cortex using (10). To decide the delay time parameter, we used the intracortical micro stimulation method (ICMS) that we shocked nine locations of the primary motor cortex 275 times by electricity, and searched the time that the EMG signals are occurred. As a result, the delay time was 16.57 ± 3.46 ms. So, we set to 17 ms. when we estimate the filtered EMG signals from the neural activities of the primary motor cortex.

Figure 11 represents the result of estimation from the neural activities to the filtered EMG signals. The estimated filtered EMG signals have a correlation coefficient of 0.93 with the actual EMG signals.

Estimation of Joint Angles from Filtered EMG Signals

To estimate joint angles from the filtered EMG signals, we used a modular artificial neural network [26], as shown in Fig. 12. Training the data of posture and movement in different network will improve the accuracy of the estimation of joint angles as compared to training the whole data in the same network since the muscle tension is different in the two mentioned cases. If training is done well, gating network

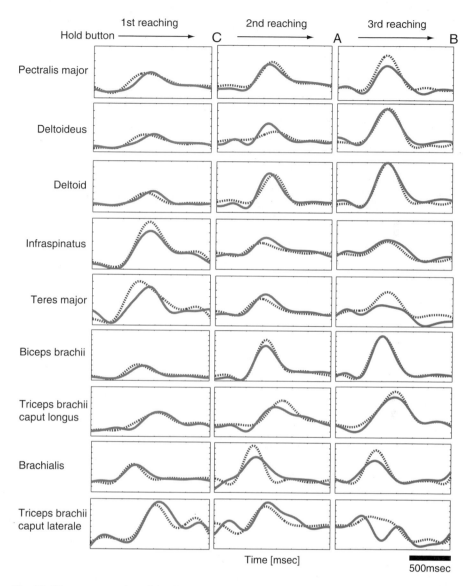

Fig. 11 The reconstruction of the filtered EMG signals using the ensemble of 105 neurons of the primary motor cortex. The *dotted lines* represent the actual filtered EMG signals and the *solid lines* show the reconstructed filtered EMG signals (color online)

selects one of two expert networks by its input signal. In this case, among two expert networks, one is for posture and another is for movement. Since the gating network decides the output ratio for each expert network depending on its input signal, the sum of the outputs of the gating network should always be 1.

The filtered EMG signals of nine muscles were used as the input of each expert network model. And, the summed squared velocity value of four joint angles was

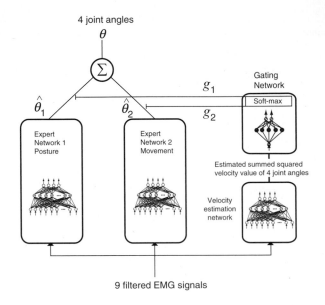

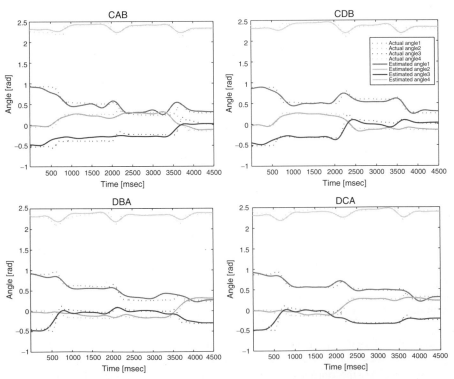

Fig. 12 Joint angle estimation model which has a modular architecture. The estimated joint angles from the neural activity of M1. *The dashed line* represents the actual joint angles and the *solid line shows* the estimated joint angles (color online)

used as the input of the gating network. When the value of the neural activities in M1 was directly used as the input of the gating network, the gating network could not distinguish the moment between posture and movement. However, when using the summed squared velocity value of four joint angles as the input, the gating network distinguished the moment of posture and movement correctly. After measuring 30 trials of the EMG signals and movement trajectories of the arm of the monkey, we used 29 trials as training data and one trial as test data. The number of training data is 522,348 samples ($29 trials \times 1$ kHz $\times 4.503$ s $\times 4 cases$) and the number of test data is 18,012 samples ($1 trial \times 1$ kHz $\times 4.503$ s $\times 4 cases$). In the case of gating network, the network was trained by the summed squared velocity value of four joint angles. However, since the summed squared velocity value of four joint angles cannot be used as test data, we estimated the velocity values of four joint angles from the filtered EMG signals. Figure 12 represents the estimated four joint angles from the neural activity of the primary motor cortex. The correlation coefficient between the estimated joint angles and the actual joint angles was about 0.92.

BCI

Conventional BCI uses EEG signals which are measured under stationary state. However, another biological signals are contaminated in EEG signal by eye movement, eye brink, heart beat, or another muscle activities. Our BCI system uses this kind noise signals for estimating movement.

Before the implementation of the system, simple experiment was made to test the feasibility and ability of classification of the eye movements. This was performed with Biosemi Active Two system, using 64 electrodes placed according to the international 10/20 system, reference electrode being placed on the left mastoid. During the experiment, eight directions were used. The subject sat in a chair, following orders displayed on a computer screen. For each sample, a fixation cross followed by an arrow was shown. Arrow being displayed, subject would move his eyes towards the direction, holding them as far as he could until the arrow was changed back into a fixation cross. This took 2 s. One hundred and sixty samples (20 for each direction) were recorded using a sampling frequency of 256 Hz. Samples were loaded into MathWorks Matlab R2007b, down sampled into 64 Hz and scaled using a moving average filter with a length of a sample length. To test the significance of the electrodes used, samples were classified with linear discriminant analysis (LDA), using the information of only one channel at a time. For a more generalized result, fourfold cross validation was used, each time training with one fourth of data. The results can be seen in Fig. 13. According to the result, producing highest results, the electrodes placed on the forehead are the most significant when detecting eye movements. Three channels are corresponded to AF7, Fpz and AF8 of the international 10/20 system.

Subjects were seated in front of a 15.4″ laptop computer according to the setting in Fig. 14. The position of the laptop monitor was adjusted to the level of eye and in the middle of the visual field so that the distance between the subjects' eyes and the

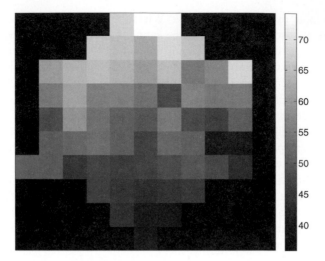

Fig. 13 Results of fourfold cross validation for all classes, using only one channel at a time. *Top* of the picture represents the front of the cap, electrodes on the forehead being the ones on the *top* of the picture

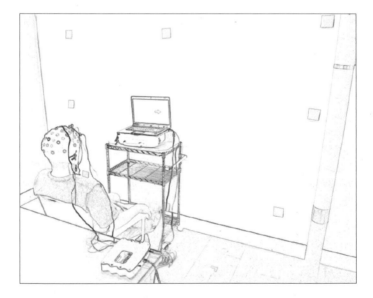

Fig. 14 Arrangement during the experiments

laptop monitor was 110 cm. After this eight markers representing the directions (right, up-right, up, up-left, left, down-left, down, down-right) were placed on a wall behind the computer so that each of them was at the edge of the limit where both eyes can fixate to. In order to do this, subjects were asked to close one of their eyes at a time and give instructions on the location for the markers. For example, one the case

Fig. 15 Structure of a set used during the training sequence

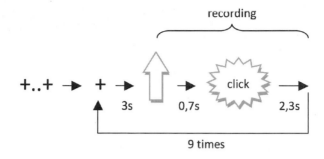

of the left marker, subject would close his left eye and point the leftmost position he could see. However the positions were kept so that the up/down markers would be in the middle along with the laptop monitor, right/left markers being at the height of the monitor and the right and left side would be symmetric to each other.

Event thought a human eye has been shown to be able to move from the middle position between 45 and 40 degrees to the sides and downwards and between 40 and 45 degrees upwards, in the preliminary tests a movement this long was noticed to be straining and eventually cause eyes to become very tired. Because of this, subjects were encouraged to choose a position slightly inwards from the limit, the angle for the subjects averaging 43 degrees to the side, 38 degrees up and 39 degrees downwards.

The experiments consisted of a training period followed with live test aimed to measure the performance of the system. During the training, eight sets each consisting of nine samples representing the different classes were recorded. Between each set, there was a 10 s brake and in addition in the middle of the training period a 30 s break took place. To inform a subject, at the beginning and at the end of a break, a sound was played. Each set consisted of two warning blinks followed by a fixation cross, a large and clear arrow indicating the direction, after which a short click sound was played. The subjects were asked to focus on the fixation cross until at the moment of an arrow shown, switch their point of gaze rapidly to a corresponding marker and when hearing the click sound, move their eyes back to the center position. During the training period, subjects were asked to refrain from blinking during the recording or if not possible, wait till the fixation cross. Per each sample, starting from the moment of the arrow was shown, 3 s of data was recorded. Including the breaks, training lasted approximately 10 min. Structure of a set is clarified in Fig. 15.

Shortly after the training, subjects were asked to briefly test the quality of the training data by systematically using all of the directions, trying their functionality in a clockwise manner. During this, subjects performed both "rounds" with and without using the center direction in between of the other directions. During the live test, to demonstrate and to test the systems functionality, a subject was asked to move a ball through a simple obstacle track using the same movements as during the training. Time was not limited and the track was designed to allow a subject to make mistakes and freely select the route. The ball would move two steps to classified direction per each 2 s sample. In addition to the movement of the ball, in order for the subject to be able to prevent performing the movement on the edge of a sample, a small click sound to help with the timing was again used between the samples.

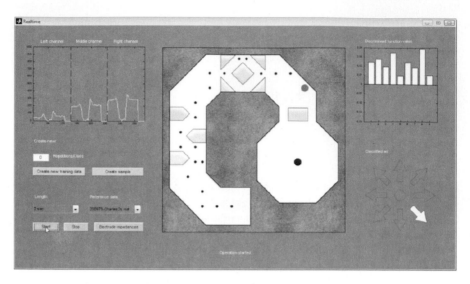

Fig. 16 The interface used during the live test. Subject is controlling the *grey ball* (actually *red*), *black dots* represent earlier positions. Also the previous feature vector, discriminant function values for the classes and the classification results can be seen

Finishing the track using the fastest route, in case of no errors, required 23 movements. The picture of the interface used can be seen in Fig. 16.

The classification is performed using multiclass LDA. Assuming that the classes have both multivariate normal distribution and same covariance matrix.

To measure the performance, the accuracy of the classification algorithm was calculated classifying both subjects data separately. This was done using 50% of the data (first four sets) for training, the rest being classified. One of the subjects did this test twice, performing six and eight sets. Accuracy was respectively 92.6 and 91.7%. Second subject performed full eight sets once, accuracy being 94.4%. During the testing of the directions functionality, one of the subjects could perform full "rounds" both with and without using the center direction in between of the other directions without having any false classifications. The classification also proved to be quite robust against eye blinks even in the case of center direction which consists mainly from noise.

Conclusion

Where Do We Have to Measure

From the computational viewpoint, one of the central issues in motor control is how arm reaching trajectories are planned. The target position is represented in Cartesian coordinates, and the muscle tension is needed for the reaching movement.

To make a plan of the movement, there are many processes that take place from decision to action, including coordinate transformations and motor command generation [27, 28]. Neural correlates of these processes are reflected in activity in the motor related cortex.

For example, the ventral premotor area (PMv) is a major source of input to M1 [29, 30]. Many PMv neurons encode the direction of movement in space. These results were strikingly different from results from M1 [31, 32]. Also, stimulation of the supplementary motor area (SMA) cell produces first an 'urge to move,' then the corresponding movement [33] or SMA cells which correspond to the elements in a sequence of movements activate during movement preparation [34]. Activities of SMA, PM and M1 play a different role in action control [35, 36]. The primary motor cortex is connected to the spinal cord either directly or via only a small number of synapses, and these motor neurons send the commands to the muscles. While SMA or PM may be the region for eliciting the intention, M1 is one of the best regions to reconstruct movement or force based on the muscle tension.

Computational Model

Knock-out mouse produce abnormal behavior by gene alteration. A target gene is mutated by the type of diseases. However, we don't know the role of genes fully, so we observe the abnormal behavior and estimate the causality.

Computational model estimates abnormal behaviour through changing gain or connection of each parts of the model which correspond to the change of neuron activities in the brain. If the behaviour is similar to the pathological condition, the change of the model might be the cause of disease. Moreover, this change may occur in the brain and it will assist the design of new physiological experiments. BMI technique based on computational model is quite valuable for not only patients and also neuroscientist so that knock-out mouse plays crucial role.

References

1. Chapin JK, Moxon KA, Markowitz RS, Nicolelis MAL (1999) Real-time control of a robot arm using simultaneously recorded neurons in the motor cortex. Nat Neurosci 2:664–670
2. Carmena JM, Lebedev MA, Crist RE, O'Doherty JE, Santucci DM, Dimitrov DF, Patil PG, Henriquez CS, Nicolelis MAL (2003) Learning to control a brain–machine interface for reaching and grasping by primates. PLoS Biol 1(2):1–16
3. Musallam S, Corneil BD, Greger B, Scherberger H, Andersen RA (2004) Cognitive control signals for neural prosthetics. Science 305(5681):258–262
4. Hochberg LR, Serruya MD, Friehs GM, Mukand JA, Saleh M, Caplan AH, Branner A, Chen D, Penn RD, Donoghue JP (2006) Neuronal ensemble control of prosthetic devices by a human with tetraplegia. Nature 442(7099):164–171
5. Georgopoulos AP, Kalaska JF, Caminiti R, Massey JT (1982) On the relations between the direction of two-dimensional arm movements and cell discharge in primate motor cortex. J Neurosci 2(11):1527–1537

6. Fetz EE, Cheney PD, German DC (1976) Corticomotoneuronal connections of precentral cells detected by postspike averages of emg activity in behaving monkeys. Brain Res 114(3):505–510
7. Kalaska JF, Cohen DA, Hyde ML, Prud'homme M (1989) A comparison of movement direction-related versus load direction-related activity in primate motor cortex, using a two-dimensional reaching task. J Neurosci 9(6):2080–2102
8. Koike Y, Kawato M (1994) Estimation of arm posture in {3D}-space from surface EMG signals using a neural network model. IEICE Trans Fundam E77-D, No. 4:368–375
9. Koike Y, Kawato M (1995) Estimation of dynamic joint torques and trajectory formation from surface electromyography signals using a neural network model. Biol Cybern 73:291–300
10. Kim J, Sato M, Koike Y (2002) Human arm posture control using the impedance controllability of the musculo-skeletal system against the alteration of the environments. Trans Control Autom Syst Eng 4(1):43–48
11. Feldman AG, Adamovich SV, Ostry DJ, Flanagan JR (1990) The origin of electromyograms – explanations based on the equilibrium point hypotheses. In: Winters JM, Woo SL-Y (eds) Multiple muscle systems. Springer, New York, pp 195–213
12. Flanagan JR, Ostry DJ, Feldman AG (1993) Control of trajectory modifications in target-directed reaching. J Mot Behav 25(3):140–152
13. Katayama M, Kawato M (1993) Virtual trajectory and stiffness ellipse during multijoint arm movement predicted by neural inverse models. Biol Cybern 69(5/6):353–362
14. Gribble PL, Ostry DJ, Sanguineti V, Laboissiere R (1998) Are complex control signals required for human arm movement? J Neurophysiol 79(3):1409–1424
15. Osu R, Gomi H (1999) Multijoint muscle regulation mechanisms examined by measured human arm stiffness and emg signals. J Neurophysiol 81:1458–1468
16. Prilutsky BI (2000) Coordination of two- and one-joint muscles: functional consequences and implications for motor control. Mot Control 4(1):1–44
17. Ghez C (2000) Principles of neural science, chapter Muscles: effectors of the motor systems. McGraw-Hill, New York
18. Özkaya N, Nordin M (1991) Fundamentals of biomechanics: equilibrium, motion, and deformation. Van Nostrand Reinhold, New York
19. Kawato M, Gomi H (1993) The cerebellum and VOR/OKR learning models. Trends Neurosci 16(11):177–178
20. Inman VT, Ralston HJ, Saunders JB, Feinstein B, Wright EW Jr (1952) Relation of human electromyogram to muscular tension. Electroencephalogr Clin Neurophysiol 4(2):187–194
21. Gottlieb GL, Agarwal GC (1971) Dynamic relationship between isometric muscle tension and the electromyogram in man. J Appl Physiol 30(3):345–351
22. Basmajian JV, De Luca CJ (1985) Description and analysis of the EMG signal. Williams & Wilkins, Baltimore, MD
23. Maton B, Peres G, Landjerit B (1987) Relationships between individual isometric muscle forces, emg activity and joint torque in monkeys. Eur J Appl Physiol Occup Physiol 56(4):487–494
24. Clancy EA, Hogan N (1991) Estimation of joint torque from the surface EMG. Annu Int Conf IEEE Eng Med Biol Soc 13(2):0877–0878
25. Choi K, Hirose H, Sakurai Y, Iijima T, Koike Y (2009) Prediction of arm trajectory from the neural activities of the primary motor cortex with modular connectionist architecture. Neural Netw 22(9):1214–1223
26. Jacobs RA, Jordan MI (1991) A competitive modular connectionist architecture. In: Moody JM, Hanson SJ, Lippmann RP (eds) Advances in neural information processing systems 3. Morgan Kaufmann, San Meteo, pp 767–773
27. Kawato M (1999) Internal models for motor control and trajectory planning. Curr Opin Neurobiol 9(6):718–727
28. Cohen YE, Andersen RA (2002) A common reference frame for movement plans in the posterior parietal cortex. Nat Rev Neurosci 3(7):553–562

29. Matsumura M, Kubota K (1979) Cortical projection of hand-arm motor area from post-arcuate area in macaque monkey: a histological study of retrograde transport of horseradish peroxidase. Neurosci Lett 11:241–246
30. Muakkassa KF, Strick PL (1979) Frontal lobe inputs to primate motor cortex: evidence for four somatotopically organized premotor areas. Brain Res 177:176–182
31. Kakei S, Hoffman DS, Strick PL (1999) Muscle and movement representations in the primary motor cortex. Science 285(5436):2136–2139
32. Kakei S, Hoffman DS, Strick PL (2001) Direction of action is represented in the ventral premotor cortex. Nat Neurosci 4(10):1020–1025
33. Fried I, Katz A, McCarthy G, Sass KJ, Williamson P, Spencer SS, Spencer DD (1991) Functional organization of human supplementary motor cortex studied by electrical stimulation. J Neurosci 11:3656–3666
34. Shima K, Tanji J (1994) Role for supplementary motor area cells in planning several movements ahead. Nature 371:413–416
35. Roland PE, Larsen B, Lassen NA, Skinhoj E (1980) Supplementary motor area and other cortical areas in organization of voluntary movements in man. J Neurophysiol 43(1):118–136
36. Halsband U, Matsuzaka Y, Tanji J (1994) Neuronal activity in the primate supplementary, presupplementary and premotor cortex during externally and internally instructed sequential movements. Neurosci Res 20(2):149–155

Improvement of Spastic Stroke Hemiparesis Using rTMS Combined with Motor Training

Satoko Koganemaru, Tatsuya Mima, Hidenao Fukuyama,
and Kazuhisa Domen

Abstract Stroke is the second most common cause of death and the leading cause of chronic disability in adults worldwide. Patients with chronic stroke often show increased flexor hypertonia in their affected upper limbs. Although an intervention strategy targeting the extensors of the affected upper limb might thus be expected to have benefits for functional recovery, conventional repetitive motor training has limited clinical utility. Recent studies have shown that repetitive transcranial magnetic stimulation (rTMS) could induce motor recovery. Therefore, we developed a new hybrid rehabilitation comprised of rTMS and motor training of the extensors in order to counteract flexor hypertonia. Five hertz rTMS of the upper-limb area of the primary motor cortex (M1), combined with extensor motor training, had a greater effect on motor recovery than either intervention alone in chronic stroke hemiparesis. It resulted in an improvement of extensor movement and grip power, along with a reduction of flexor hypertonia in their paretic upper limbs. In addition, we found the long-lasting effect for more than 2 weeks, by repeating the hyprid rehabilitation 12 times in patients for 6 weeks. These findings indicate that this method can facilitate use-dependent plasticity and achieve functional recovery of motor impairments. This new hybrid form of rehabilitation could be a powerful rehabilitative approach for patients with hemiparetic stroke.

S. Koganemaru (✉)
Human Brain Research Center, Kyoto University School of Medicine,
54, Shogoin Kawahara-cho, Sakyo-ku, Kyoto 606-8507, Japan
and
Department of Physical and Rehabilitation Medicine, Hyogo College of Medicine,
1-1, Mukogawa-cho, Nishinomiya, Hyogo 663-8501, Japan
e-mail: kogane@kuhp.kyoto-u.ac.jp

T. Mima (✉) • H. Fukuyama
Human Brain Research Center, Kyoto University School of Medicine,
54, Shogoin Kawahara-cho, Sakyo-ku, Kyoto 606-8507, Japan
e-mail: mima@kuhp.kyoto-u.ac.jp

K. Domen
Department of Physical and Rehabilitation Medicine, Hyogo College of Medicine,
1-1, Mukogawa-cho, Nishinomiya, Hyogo 663-8501, Japan

K. Kansaku and L.G. Cohen (eds.), *Systems Neuroscience and Rehabilitation*,
DOI 10.1007/978-4-431-54008-3_4, © Springer 2011

Neuroplasticity After Stroke

Stroke is the second most common cause of death and the leading cause of chronic disability in adults worldwide [1]. After the onset of ischaemic insult, the brain starts to reorganize itself. Plastic changes have been demonstrated in cerebral cortex and in subcortical structures at the synaptic, cellular, and network level. In vitro studies, oxygen and glucose deprivation (in vitro ischemia) exerts long-term effects on the efficacy of synaptic transmission via the induction of a post-ischemic long-term potentiation (i-LTP). i-LTP may deeply influence the plastic reorganization of cortical representational maps, through strengthening synaptic connection with residual neurons and generating a new functional connection of previously non-interacting neurons, while it may exert detrimental effects on neuronal cells through its excitotoxicity [2]. Human stroke patients showed that various cortical areas in bilateral hemispheres were activated in imaging and electrophysiological studies [3, 4]. On the process of motor recovery, decreased activities were found in primary motor cortex (M1), premotor and prefrontal cortex, supplementary motor areas, cingulate sulcus, temporal lobe, striate cortex, cerebellum, thalamus and basal ganglia, independent of rate of recovery or initial severity of stroke patients [4]. Recovery usually occurred during around 1–12 weeks after the onset [5–7]. Rehabilitative intervention in this acute and subacute phases is considered to be very important, which facilitates brain reorganization leading to functional recovery. Nudo et al. showed that after an infarct of M1 hand area of adult squirrel monkeys, retraining of skilled hand use resulted in prevention of the loss of hand area adjacent to the infarct site by expanding it into elbow and shoulder area [8]. In humans, a randomized controlled trial showed the structured, progressive program of therapeutic exercise in acute rehabilitation services, produced gains in endurance, balance and mobility beyond those attributable to spontaneous recovery and usual care in stroke patients [9]. Therefore, traditional rehabilitation is considered as one of the therapeutic tools to augment the post-stroke recovery process.

However, later in the chronic phase, there is little probability of spontaneous neuroplastic changes. In the time course of post-stroke motor recovery, no significant improvement has been found later than 6 months after the onset [10, 11]. The most striking improvements of the functional ability of arm, trunk and leg were found from 1 week to 1 month, without any improvements between 3 and 6 months [11]. A valid prognosis of upper extremity function could be made within 3 and 6 weeks, and any further recovery could not be found after 6 and 11 weeks in patients with mild and severe paresis, respectively [10].

Furthermore, maladaptive neuroplastic changes may occur in chronic phase. For example, we may observe the learned non-use of the paretic limb which can worsen the residual function or the over-suppression of the affected hemisphere due to imbalanced interhemispheric inhibitory system [12].

Therefore, our rehabilitation goal is to induce neural plasticity which facilitates functional recovery and which corrects the maladaptive one.

Strategies for Recovery in Chronic Stroke: Intensive Motor Therapy and Non-Invasive Brain Stimulation

Recent reports suggested that functional recovery might occur even in chronic patients if plastic changes are induced by intense motor training or non-invasive cortical stimulation. Constraint-induced movement therapy (CIMT) is one of the successful approaches for paretic upper limbs in chronic stroke patients. It was derived from basic research with monkeys given somatosensory deafferentation and is based on a behavioral theory of 'learned non-use' of the affected limb [13]. It is considered to be effective because it reverses the learned non-use condition with two main components: (1) constraining the movement of the healthy upper extremity, and (2) intensive training of the paretic arm. It was shown to be effective in a subset of stroke patients with mild hemiparesis, who could exert some extension of a wrist and fingers [14–16]. Along with improvements of motor performance after CIMT, dynamic brain reorganization was demonstrated at cortical and subcortical level [17–19]. There was an increase of size of motor output area and motor-evoked potential (MEP) amplitudes, indicating enhanced neuronal excitability in the damaged hemisphere for the target muscles. The mean center of gravity of the motor output maps was shifted considerably, indicating the recruitment of motor areas adjacent to the original location [19]. In neuroimaging studies, there was a linear reduction in ipsilateral (contralesional) M1 activation (voxel counts) across time. The change in ipsilateral M1 voxel count correlated with the improvements of motor performance [17]. By using the imaging technique of voxel based morphology, the structural changes such as increases or decreases in amount of gray matter concentration paralleled the improvements in spontaneous use of the impaired arm in activities of daily living after CIMT. There were profuse increases in gray matter concentration in sensory and motor areas both contralateral and ipsilateral to the affected arm that were bilaterally symmetrical, as well as bilaterally in the hippocampus. Importantly, the magnitude of those increases was significantly correlated with amount of improvement in real-world arm use [18].

Non-invasive cortical stimulation such as transcranial magnetic stimulation (TMS) and transcranial direct current stimulation (tDCS) has been proposed to modulate neural plasticity, enhance it when it plays an adaptive role, and down-regulate it when it is considered maladaptive. That is, LTP-like effects of high-frequency repetitive TMS (rTMS) or anodal stimulation of tDCS can be given to the affected hemisphere to produce functional facilitation by increasing the cortical excitability, while LTD-like effects of low-frequency rTMS or cathodal stimulation of rDCS can be applied to suppress the intact hemisphere to produce the functional facilitation of the affected side through the decrease of interhemispheric inhibition [12]. When high-frequency rTMS was given over M1 in the affected side daily for 10 days, patients with acute stroke showed improvements of disability scales at the end of the last rTMS session, which lasts at least 10 days [20]. After 10 Hz rTMS over the affected M1, chronic stroke patients showed enhanced accuracy of motor performance in a complex, sequential finger motor task using their paretic fingers, in addition to a significantly larger increase in the MEP amplitude [21]. Anodal tDCS given over the M1 in the affected hemisphere improved hand functions that mimic activities of daily living in the paretic hand of chronic stroke patients, correlated with an increment in motor cortical excitability within the affected hemisphere and reduced short-interval intracortical inhibition. Its effects outlasted the stimulation period. It suggested that tDCS may play an adjuvant role in combination with customary rehabilitative treatments [22]. Therefore, high-frequency rTMS or anodal tDCS to the affected motor cortex is considered to facilitate use-dependent plasticity (UDP) and to improve the motor learning performance in stroke patients.

On the other hand, low-frequency rTMS or cathodal tDCS to the intact hemisphere decreases interhemispheric inhibition from the intact hemisphere to the affected one, leading to functional improvement in stroke hemiparetic patients. Motor performance such as reaction time or the Purdue Pegboard test was significantly improved in their affected hand [23]. An improvement in pinch acceleration of the affected hand was accompanied with the reduced MEP amplitudes and transcallosal inhibition in the intact M1. The improvements were significantly correlated with reduction of transcallosal inhibition [24]. The long-term beneficial effects are confirmed by repeating rTMS sessions. Five sessions of low-frequency rTMS could increase the magnitude and duration of these effects, resulting in a significant improvement of the motor performance with the affected hand, which lasted for 2 weeks. There was a significant correlation between motor functional improvement and increases of corticospinal excitability in the affected hemisphere [25]. After cathodal tDCS over the intact hemisphere, a significant improvement was also found in motor performance in the paretic hands. Consecutive daily sessions of cathodal tDCS lasted the effects for 2 weeks [26].

A new stimulation protocol of rTMS, theta burst stimulation which can produce consistent effects on the cortical excitability very rapidly, using lower stimulation intensity and a shorter time of stimulation [27, 28], might be also effective in chronic stroke patients. Immediately after excitatory TBS (intermittent TBS, iTBS) over the affected hemisphere, simple reaction time was significantly decreased along with increases of the MEP amplitudes and of the area under the input–output curves in the affected hemisphere. Inhibitory TBS (continuous TBS, cTBS) over the intact hemisphere suppressed the MEP amplitudes but did not change motor behaviour or the electrophysiological parameters in the affected hemisphere [29].

Although intensive motor training or non-invasive brain stimulation seems to be successful in stroke rehabilitation, their effectiveness might be limited to patients with mild hemiparesis who could exert separative movements of hands and arm [12]. Those patients might only account for one-forth of the whole stroke victims [12, 16]. In order to restore the upper limb function of stroke patients including those with moderate-to-severe hemiparesis, we might need a new powerful approach which could induce neural plasticity more efficiently.

A New Hybrid Form of Rehabilitation: Motor Training and Brain Stimulation

Patients with chronic stroke, with moderate-to-severe hemiparesis, often suffer from motor deficits associated with flexor hypertonia, as well as motor weakness. Thus, there are two possible therapeutic strategies for these patients. The first one is to develop a new method to induce LTP-like M1 plasticity as strong as possible. However, in this case, we have the risk of inducing epilepsy by using high intensity of brain stimulation [30]. Another strategy is to selectively induce LTP-like plasticity in the extensor-muscles function in order to counteract the flexor hypertonia.

In healthy subjects, use-dependent plasticity (UDP) has been reported, in which motor training induced LTP-like changes in the cortico-spinal neurons representing only agonist, but not antagonist, muscles for a trained movement [31, 32]. However, as described above, the beneficial effects of training in chronic-phase patients are relatively limited [10, 11]. Even in the subacute phase, additional extensor training of the affected hand did not change the clinical outcome [33].

To utilize UDP for stroke rehabilitation, one may combine excitatory rTMS of the M1 area for the affected side with repetitive movements of the paretic upper limb. It may be possible to achieve the selective enhancement of the trained movement, despite of the non-specific facilitatory effects of rTMS for both agonist and antagonist muscles due to its limited spatial resolution. We explored the effects of the combined intervention of high-frequency rTMS and repetitive wrist and finger extension exercises, that is, a new hybrid form of rehabilitation. Since patients with moderate-to-severe hemiparesis have difficulty in executing the voluntary repetitive movements necessary for UDP, we used neuromuscular stimulation to aid extensor training [34].

The stroke patients performed 15 cycles of exercises for the extensors of the wrist and fingers. Each cycle consisted of exercises for the extensors for 50 s followed by a train of 5 Hz repetitive TMS for 8 s, which was both preceded and followed by a resting period of 1 s (total time = 1 min) ('EEx–TMS', Fig. 1). The exercises for the extensors comprised 50 repeats of 1 Hz rhythmic voluntary extension of the wrist and metacarpophalangeal (MCP) joints of the five digits aided by electrical neuromuscular stimulation across the extensor digitorum communis (EDC) muscle, followed by brief relaxation (rather than voluntary flexion). Five hertz rTMS was performed with a coil placed in the optimal position in the M1 to elicit the best motor response in the target EDC muscles. As control experiments, we also examined the single intervention effect of the exercises with sham TMS ('EEx', Fig. 1) and the single intervention effect of the 5 Hz rTMS ('TMS', Fig. 1). To assess the effects of the interventions on behavioural parameters, and particularly to differentiate the effects of the training on agonist and antagonist muscles, clinical assessments were made of the active range of movement (ROM) for the wrist joint and the MCP joints of the thumb, index finger and middle finger both in extension and flexion in the paretic side. Pinch force and grip power were also assessed. In addition, in order to evaluate muscle hypertonia, we measured the changes of the modified Ashworth scale (mAS) scores [35, 36].

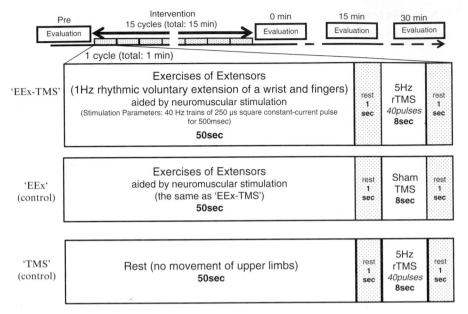

Fig. 1 Experimental paradigm. In the main experiment ('EEx–TMS', *upper*), 15 cycles of focal extensor exercises ('EEx'), consisting of 1 Hz rhythmic voluntary movements of the wrist and fingers aided or triggered by neuromuscular stimulation of the EDC muscles, were combined with high-frequency repetitive TMS ('TMS'). Each cycle consisted of exercises for the extensors for 50 s followed by a train of 5 Hz repetitive TMS for 8 s, which was both preceded and followed by a resting period of 1 s (total time = 1 min). In the control experiments, exercises for the extensors combined with sham TMS ('EEx': *middle*) or 5 Hz repetitive TMS alone ('TMS': *lower*) were used. Motor functions (behavioural and electrophysiological parameters in each experiment) were evaluated before, immediately after, 15 min after and 30 min after the end of the intervention (the pre, post-0, post-15 and post-30 conditions, respectively). rTMS = repetitive TMS

As a result, we found that significant increases of the active ROMs in extension for the wrist joint and MCP joints of the fingers after 'EEx–TMS', while the active ROMs in flexion were not significantly changed. The grip power in the paretic side was significantly improved and the mAS scores of the wrist joint and MCP joints of the fingers were significantly decreased, whereas there were no significant changes after 'EEx' or 'TMS' alone. The combined intervention, 'EEx–TMS', but neither of the single interventions of 'EEx' or 'TMS', resulted in an improvement of extensor movement, but not flexor one, and grip power along with a reduction of flexor hypertonia in the paretic upper limbs of stroke patients. It was likely that plasticity for the specific movements – that is, UDP – had occurred.

However, we could not evaluate electrophysiological parameters in detail for all the patients due to their elevated motor threshold of the affected limb. Therefore, we evaluated them in healthy subjects who received the same interventions of 'EEx–TMS', 'EEx' and 'TMS'.

As a result, after 'EEx–TMS', we found that the MEP amplitudes of the EDC muscles which were agonist muscles for the motor training, were significantly enhanced, while those of the flexors carpi radialis (FCR) muscles which were antagonist ones, were not. After the 'EEx', the MEP amplitudes of the EDC and FCR muscles were not significantly changed. After the 'TMS', the MEP amplitudes of the FCR muscles were significantly increased, whereas those of the EDC muscles showed a non-significant tendency to increase. For the input–output functions, significant increases of the MEP amplitude were found after 'EEx–TMS'. The other two types of session did not cause any significant changes. The resting motor threshold (rMT) of the EDC muscles was significantly decreased after 'EEx–TMS', while that of the FCR muscles was not. After the other two types of sessions, it was not significantly changed. After 'EEx–TMS', the silent period of the EDC muscles was significantly increased while that of the right FCR muscles was not. After 'EEx' and 'TMS', it was not significantly changed.

The combined intervention 'EEx–TMS' could induce UDP that was specific for agonist, but not antagonist, muscles whereas the 'TMS' intervention could influence the muscles non-specifically, and 'EEx' failed to induce any significant changes. In the M1 and the premotor area, neurons are coded for specific movement [37–40]. The results suggested that the function of neurons for specific movement (in this case, extension of the wrist and fingers) could be improved by enhanced excitability or synaptic efficacy of the appropriate neuronal population.

In order to investigate the long-lasting effects of the repeated 'EEx–TMS', we performed 12 times of 'EEx–TMS' on the stroke patients, with one session per day, on two separate days per week, for 6 weeks in total. The same assessments were done before the 12 sessions, at the end of the 12 sessions (6 weeks) and 2 weeks after the 12 sessions (8 weeks). As a result, we found significant increases of the active ROMs both in extension and flexion for the wrist joint and the MCP joints of the fingers. The pinch force and grip power in the paretic side were significantly increased after 6 and 8 weeks. Significant decreases of the mAS scores were found in the wrist joint and the MCP joints of the thumb and middle finger.

Performing the 'EEx–TMS' sessions over 6 weeks (12 times in total) induced an long-term improvement of active ROM not only in extension but also in flexion along with the reduction of flexors hypertonia. Continuing the intervention for a longer period than 6 weeks might have improved muscle contracture such as short-ened muscle fibre and stiffened connective tissues produced by the persistent non-use condition [41–44], resulting in the functional improvements of the whole upper limbs in the stroke patients.

This new hybrid form of neurorehabilitation could be a powerful approach for hemiparetic stroke patients and might be applied to patients with other various movement disorders.

So far, there have been a number of forms of rehabilitative therapy with uncer-tain results as to differences in efficacy across schools of approach. In order to determine how various rehabilitation/repair therapies have effects on recovery, translational studies are also needed. And standardized post-stroke therapy protocols need to be established and their practice associated with proper training [45]. Neurorehabilitation remains to be developed and validated.

References

1. Feigin V, Anderson N, Gunn A, Rodgers A, Anderson C (2003) The emerging role of therapeutic hypothermia in acute stroke. Lancet Neurol 2:529
2. Di Filippo M, Tozzi A, Costa C, Belcastro V, Tantucci M, Picconi B, Calabresi P (2008) Plasticity and repair in the post-ischemic brain. Neuropharmacology 55:353–362
3. Trompetto C, Assini A, Buccolieri A, Marchese R, Abbruzzese G (2000) Motor recovery following stroke: a transcranial magnetic stimulation study. Clin Neurophysiol 111:1860–1867
4. Ward NS, Brown MM, Thompson AJ, Frackowiak RS (2003) Neural correlates of motor recovery after stroke: a longitudinal fMRI study. Brain 126:2476–2496
5. Ito U, Kawakami E, Nagasao J, Kuroiwa T, Nakano I, Oyanagi K (2006) Restitution of ischemic injuries in penumbra of cerebral cortex after temporary ischemia. Acta Neurochir Suppl 96:239–243
6. Ito U, Kuroiwa T, Nagasao J, Kawakami E, Oyanagi K (2006) Temporal profiles of axon terminals, synapses and spines in the ischemic penumbra of the cerebral cortex: ultrastructure of neuronal remodeling. Stroke 37:2134–2139
7. Rossini PM, Calautti C, Pauri F, Baron JC (2003) Post-stroke plastic reorganisation in the adult brain. Lancet Neurol 2:493–502
8. Nudo RJ, Wise BM, SiFuentes F, Milliken GW (1996) Neural substrates for the effects of rehabilitative training on motor recovery after ischemic infarct. Science 272:1791–1794
9. Duncan P, Studenski S, Richards L, Gollub S, Lai SM, Reker D, Perera S, Yates J, Koch V, Rigler S, Johnson D (2003) Randomized clinical trial of therapeutic exercise in subacute stroke. Stroke 34:2173–2180
10. Nakayama H, Jorgensen HS, Raaschou HO, Olsen TS (1994) Recovery of upper extremity function in stroke patients: the Copenhagen stroke study. Arch Phys Med Rehabil 75:394–398
11. Verheyden G, Nieuwboer A, De Wit L, Thijs V, Dobbelaere J, Devos H, Severijns D, Vanbeveren S, De Weerdt W (2008) Time course of trunk, arm, leg, and functional recovery after ischemic stroke. Neurorehabil Neural Repair 22:173–179
12. Hummel FC, Cohen LG (2005) Drivers of brain plasticity. Curr Opin Neurol 18:667–674
13. Taub E (1980) Somatosensory deafferentiation research with monkeys: implications for rehabilitation medicine. In: Ince LP (ed) Behavioral psychology in rehabilitation medicine: clinical applications. Williams & Wilkins, New York
14. Taub E, Miller NE, Novack TA, Cook Iii EW, Fleming WC, Nepomuceno CS, Connell JS, Crago JE (1993) Technique to improve chronic motor deficit after stroke. Arch Phys Med Rehabil 74:347–354
15. Wolf SL, Lecraw E, Barton LA, Jann BB (1989) Forced use of hemiplegic upper extremities to reverse the effect of learned nonuse among chronic stroke and head-injured patients. Exp Neurol 104:125–132
16. Wolf SL, Winstein CJ, Miller JP, Taub E, Uswatte G, Morris D, Giuliani C, Light KE, Nichols-Larsen D (2006) Effect of constraint-induced movement therapy on upper extremity function 3 to 9 months after stroke: the EXCITE randomized clinical trial. JAMA 296:2095–2104
17. Dong Y, Dobkin BH, Cen SY, Wu AD, Winstein CJ (2006) Motor cortex activation during treatment may predict therapeutic gains in paretic hand function after stroke. Stroke 37:1552–1555
18. Gauthier LV, Taub E, Perkins C, Ortmann M, Mark VW, Uswatte G (2008) Remodeling the brain: plastic structural brain changes produced by different motor therapies after stroke * supplemental material. Stroke 39:1520–1525
19. Liepert J, Miltner WH, Bauder H, Sommer M, Dettmers C, Taub E, Weiller C (1998) Motor cortex plasticity during constraint-induced movement therapy in stroke patients. Neurosci Lett 250:5–8
20. Khedr EM, Ahmed MA, Fathy N, Rothwell JC (2005) Therapeutic trial of repetitive transcranial magnetic stimulation after acute ischemic stroke. Neurology 65:466–468
21. Kim YH, You SH, Ko MH, Park JW, Lee KH, Jang SH, Yoo WK, Hallett M (2006) Repetitive transcranial magnetic stimulation-induced corticomotor excitability and associated motor skill acquisition in chronic stroke. Stroke 37:1471–1476

22. Hummel F, Celnik P, Giraux P, Floel A, Wu W-H, Gerloff C, Cohen LG (2005) Effects of non-invasive cortical stimulation on skilled motor function in chronic stroke. Brain 128:490–499
23. Mansur CG, Fregni F, Boggio PS, Riberto M, Gallucci-Neto J, Santos CM, Wagner T, Rigonatti SP, Marcolin MA, Pascual-Leone A (2005) A sham stimulation-controlled trial of rTMS of the unaffected hemisphere in stroke patients. Neurology 64:1802–1804
24. Takeuchi N, Chuma T, Matsuo Y, Watanabe I, Ikoma K (2005) Repetitive transcranial magnetic stimulation of contralesional primary motor cortex improves hand function after stroke. Stroke 36:2681–2686
25. Fregni F, Boggio PS, Valle AC, Rocha RR, Duarte J, Ferreira MJ, Wagner T, Fecteau S, Rigonatti SP, Riberto M, Freedman SD, Pascual-Leone A (2006) A sham-controlled trial of a 5-day course of repetitive transcranial magnetic stimulation of the unaffected hemisphere in stroke patients. Stroke 37:2115–2122
26. Boggio PS, Nunes A, Rigonatti SP, Nitsche MA, Pascual-Leone A, Fregni F (2007) Repeated sessions of noninvasive brain DC stimulation is associated with motor function improvement in stroke patients. Restor Neurol Neurosci 25:123–129
27. Cardenas-Morales L, Nowak DA, Kammer T, Wolf RC, Schonfeldt-Lecuona C (2010) Mechanisms and applications of theta-burst rTMS on the human motor cortex. Brain Topogr 22:294–306
28. Huang YZ, Edwards MJ, Rounis E, Bhatia KP, Rothwell JC (2005) Theta burst stimulation of the human motor cortex. Neuron 45:201–206
29. Talelli P, Greenwood RJ, Rothwell JC (2007) Exploring theta burst stimulation as an intervention to improve motor recovery in chronic stroke. Clin Neurophysiol 118:333–342
30. Lomarev MP, Kim DY, Richardson SP, Voller B, Hallett M (2007) Safety study of high-frequency transcranial magnetic stimulation in patients with chronic stroke. Clin Neurophysiol 118:2072–2075
31. Butefisch CM, Davis BC, Sawaki L, Waldvogel D, Classen J, Kopylev L, Cohen LG (2002) Modulation of use-dependent plasticity by d-amphetamine. Ann Neurol 51:59–68
32. Butefisch CM, Davis BC, Wise SP, Sawaki L, Kopylev L, Classen J, Cohen LG (2000) Mechanisms of use-dependent plasticity in the human motor cortex. Proc Natl Acad Sci USA 97:3661–3665
33. Trombly CA, Thayer-Nason L, Bliss G, Girard CA, Lyrist LA, Brexa-Hooson A (1986) The effectiveness of therapy in improving finger extension in stroke patients. Am J Occup Ther 40:612–617
34. Koganemaru S, Mima T, Thabit MN, Ikkaku T, Shimada K, Kanematsu M, Takahashi K, Fawi G, Takahashi R, Fukuyama H, Domen K (2010) Recovery of upper-limb function due to enhanced use-dependent plasticity in chronic stroke patients. Brain 133:3373–3384
35. Ashworth B (1964) Preliminary trial of carisoprodol in multiple sclerosis. Practitioner 192:540–543
36. Bohannon RW, Smith MB (1987) Interrater reliability of a modified Ashworth scale of muscle spasticity. Phys Ther 67:206–207
37. Georgopoulos AP, Kalaska JF, Caminiti R, Massey JT (1982) On the relations between the direction of two-dimensional arm movements and cell discharge in primate motor cortex. J Neurosci 2:1527–1537
38. Kakei S, Hoffman DS, Strick PL (2001) Direction of action is represented in the ventral premotor cortex. Nat Neurosci 4:1020–1025
39. Muir RB, Lemon RN (1983) Corticospinal neurons with a special role in precision grip. Brain Res 261:312–316
40. Rizzolatti G, Fadiga L, Gallese V, Fogassi L (1996) Premotor cortex and the recognition of motor actions. Brain Res Cogn Brain Res 3:131–141
41. Akeson WH, Woo SL, Amiel D, Matthews JV (1974) Biomechanical and biochemical changes in the periarticular connective tissue during contracture development in the immobilized rabbit knee. Connect Tissue Res 2:315–323
42. Dietz V, Ketelsen UP, Berger W, Quintern J (1986) Motor unit involvement in spastic paresis. Relationship between leg muscle activation and histochemistry. J Neurol Sci 75:89–103

43. Edstrom L (1970) Selective changes in the sizes of red and white muscle fibres in upper motor lesions and Parkinsonism. J Neurol Sci 11:537–550
44. Goldspink G, Tabary C, Tabary JC, Tardieu C, Tardieu G (1974) Effect of denervation on the adaptation of sarcomere number and muscle extensibility to the functional length of the muscle. J Physiol 236:733–742
45. Hachinski V, Donnan GA, Gorelick PB, Hacke W, Cramer SC, Kaste M, Fisher M, Brainin M, Buchan AM, Lo EH, Skolnick BE, Furie KL, Hankey GJ, Kivipelto M, Morris J, Rothwell PM, Sacco RL, Smith SC Jr, Wang Y, Bryer A, Ford GA, Iadecola C, Martins SCO, Saver J, Skvortsova V, Bayley M, Bednar MM, Duncan P, Enney L, Finklestein S, Jones TA, Kalra L, Kleim J, Nitkin R, Teasell R, Weiller C, Desai B, Goldberg MP, Heiss W-D, Saarelma O, Schwamm LH, Shinohara Y, Trivedi B, Wahlgren N, Wong LK, Hakim A, Norrving B, Prudhomme S, Bornstein NM, Davis SM, Goldstein LB, Leys D, Tuomilehto J (2010) Stroke: working toward a prioritized world agenda. Stroke 41:1084–1099

Molecular and Electrophysiological Approaches for Functional Recovery in Patients with Injured Spinal Cord

Toru Ogata, Noritaka Kawashima, Kimitaka Nakazawa, and Masami Akai

Abstract Because patients with an injured spinal cord face severe functional deficits, novel therapeutic approaches are required to treat this traumatic disorder. Recent advances in molecular biology and electrophysiology have rendered approaches based on these two subjects important in this field. A molecular approach involving tissue engineering is beneficial for preserving or restoring the neural circuit, i.e., the so-called "hardware" of the spinal cord. On the other hand, the electrophysiological approach has advantages such as modulation and analysis of use-dependent plastic changes in neural functioning of human subjects, which corresponds to the "software" of the spinal cord. Because varied biological processes are triggered after spinal cord injury, we should use either approach, or both, depending on the clinical problem that needs to be solved.

Hardware and Software of Spinal Cord Injury

In Japan, about 4,000 new cases of spinal cord injury (SCI) have been reported. Because of advances in medical treatment for the acute and chronic phase of this traumatic disorder, the mortality rate among patients with SCI has declined. However, there are increasing numbers of patients with SCI who face severe sensory and motor functional deficits for the rest of their lives. Therefore, the development of novel therapeutic approaches for functional recovery of patients with SCI is essential for not only the patients and their families but also for socio-economic reasons.

T. Ogata (✉) · N. Kawashima · K. Nakazawa · M. Akai
Department of Rehabilitation for Movement Functions,
Research Institute of National Rehabilitation Center for Persons with Disabilities (NRCD),
4-1 Namiki, Tokorozawa, Saitama 359-8555, Japan
e-mail: ogata-toru@rehab.go.jp

K. Kansaku and L.G. Cohen (eds.), *Systems Neuroscience and Rehabilitation*,
DOI 10.1007/978-4-431-54008-3_5, © Springer 2011

Because SCI triggers complicated biological processes and also leads to a variety of neuronal deficits, the use of several approaches should be considered. The approaches can be categorized into the "hardware" and "software" approach. "Hardware" implies the neural network through which all neural activities take place. Just as a computer does not work unless a suitable program is installed, the neural "hardware" also requires neural programs that control limbs and coordinate movement. In the neural network, such programs include proper synaptic connections, which facilitate basic voluntary movement of the limbs and learning of complex motor patterns. Traumatic disturbance in the neural circuit leads to the simultaneous reorganization and reprogramming of the neural circuit. With regard to therapeutic intervention, the "hardware" approach would entail pharmacological therapy for neuroprotection in patients with acute phase SCI or it would entail tissue engineering for the restoration of the neural structure. On the other hand, rehabilitation and training, which facilitate use-dependent plasticity, are regarded as "software" approaches (Fig. 1).

The molecular and electrophysiological approaches both can be used for analysis of nervous system disorders and therapeutic intervention. The molecular approach is based on the knowledge of molecular cellular biology and aiming to modulate cellular functions in patients with SCI. For example, cell death modulation and apoptosis are closely related to the prevention of secondary injury, which is reported to be a main cause of progressive damage in patients with acute phase SCI. In the same manner, basic research on axonal elongation revealed the existence of inhibitory factors

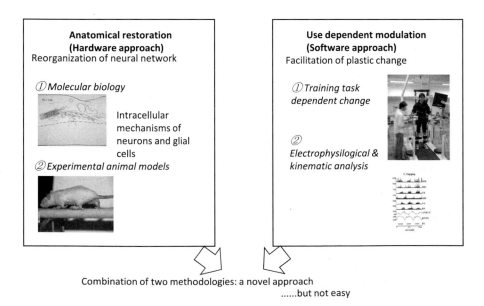

Combination of two methodologies: a novel approach
......but not easy

Fig. 1 Two methodologies for intervention in spinal cord injury. There are molecular approaches (*left*) and electrophysiological approaches (*right*) for analyzing and biological processes after SCI and providing therapeutic intervention

such as Nogo in the injured spinal cord, which acts on a group of receptors that induce the growth cone shrinkage leading to the termination of axonal regeneration. Now, this molecular mechanism is regarded as a therapeutic target to induce axonal regeneration, and various pharmacological approaches based on this are now in the preclinical stages of investigation. Taken together, the molecular approach is thought to be an effective means of modifying the neural structure (hardware).

On the other hand, the electrophysiological approach is effective in measuring or modulating neural functions. Various noninvasive means such as electromyography, measurement of nerve conduction velocity, and transcranial magnetic stimulation are used to assess the connectivity of supraspinal circuits and distal neural circuits, and the excitabilities of the corticospinal tract in human subjects. Recently, it is also used as a method to modify neural activities in the central nervous system through the use of transcranial magnetic stimulation or transcranial direct current stimulation. Therefore, these methods are effective in detecting or inducing plastic change in neural activities, which is related to "software."

To establish a multidisciplinary approach to SCI, it would be interesting to combine those approaches, so that the basic knowledge of molecular biology can be applied directly to a clinical setting. However, there have not been many models that have been used successfully for this purpose probably because of the unavailability of a proper animal spinal cord injury model for observing plastic change in neural activity in an electrophysiological manner. Therefore, at this point, it would be better to utilize either of the two methodologies depending on the clinical problem that needs to be solved.

Approaches for Treating Complete Spinal Cord Injury

Patients with SCI show varied symptoms and levels of severity. With regard to severity, there is (1) complete SCI, i.e., complete loss of sensory and motor functions below the lesion, and there is also (2) incomplete SCI, i.e., preservation of sensory and motor functions. In the case of complete SCI, especially in patients with severe dislocation of the spinal column, the connection between the brain and lower circuits seems to be completely lost. In such cases, it is important to restore some connection beyond the lesion before considering reprogramming the reorganized neural circuits. For this purpose, the molecular approach has an advantage over the electrophysiological approach.

As mentioned above, molecular biology has revealed much about the mechanisms governing axonal elongation. Especially, the intracellular mechanisms that are triggered by nerve growth factor stimuli have been investigated in detail. Nerve growth factors (NGFs), brain-derived neurotrophic factor (BDNF), and neurotrophin-3 (NT-3) bind to their own receptors expressed on the cell surface of neurons and transduce their effects via phosphorylation cascades of signaling molecules within the cell, which finally induce gene expression for axonal elongation. Among several signaling cascades, activation of the Mek–Erk signals is said to be important, and it has been shown that Mek activation is sufficient to induce axonal growth in PC12 cell line – a model cell line for neurite growth – even in the absence of nerve growth factors. Miura et al. examined the application of this paradigm in a spinal cord injury model [1]. In their report, he transected rat spinal cord at the thoracic 10 level and injected an adenovirus gene transfer vector into the parenchyma of the proximal stump. This type of gene transfer delivered the gene to not only the segmental neural cells in the spinal cord but also the primary motor neurons in the brain, such as the red nucleus, by retrograde transport along the axons. After 6 weeks of spinal transection and simultaneous gene transfer of the control gene (LacZ) or the constitutively active *Mek* gene, the effect of gene transfer was examined by both behavioral and histological evaluation. Behavioral evaluation using the Basso, Beattie, and Bresnahan (BBB) scale [2], which has been a well-accepted hind limb motor scoring scale in a rat spinal cord injury model, showed better functional recovery in the active Mek-transferred group than in the control group (Fig. 2). Histological evaluation performed by injecting an anterograde neuronal-tracer into the red nucleus

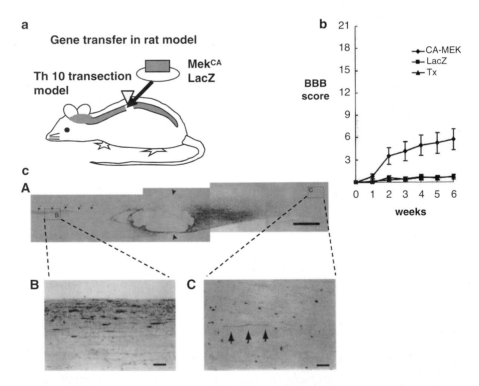

Fig. 2 A molecular approach for treating complete SCI. For complete SCI, we have shown the restoration of axonal connectivity between the supra-spinal circuit and the area below the lesion. (**a**) Schematic image of the transfer of a gene to the transected spinal cord using adenoviral vectors. (**b**) Functional recovery was observed in the CA-MEK transferred group, in which the intracellular MEK–ERK signaling cascade is constitutively activated in primary motor neurons of the brain. (**c**) Histological examination reveals axonal regeneration beyond the lesion (anterograde neurotracing)

showed marked regeneration of the rubrospinal tract beyond the complete transection site. Taken together, activation of intracellular signals within the primary motor neuron in the brain can be one of the approaches to retain functional recovery in cases in which the axonal connection is completely lost at the lesion site.

Approaches for Treating Incomplete Spinal Cord Injury

The therapeutic strategy for patients with incomplete SCI should be different from that for those with complete SCI. Because the symptoms for this condition are varied and the degree of severity and the segment injured varies among patients with incomplete SCI, the patient's condition needs to be thoroughly investigated, and the aspect of neural function that requires treatment should be determined. For example, the treatment approach for a patient who cannot stand even with support should differ from that for one who can walk with support but with a spastic gait. Here, we will discuss gait rehabilitation in patients with incomplete SCI, especially those who can stand with assistive tools and walk a few steps with assistance. These patients are classified as Frankel C and are considered to probably have SCI of "mild" severity. However, it is not practical for these patients to perform loco-motion activity.

With regard to the modification of neural functions, physiological functions should be strengthened; and abnormal functions, corrected. Besides facilitation of voluntary movement of the lower limbs, automated movement of limbs is also con-sidered an important physiological neural function in those patients. While walking, individuals do not have to pay attention to how to move their hip, knee, and ankle joints. It has been shown that a certain "gait program" exists within the central ner-vous systems and that we utilize this program. The existence of the gait program is shown using an experimental model of decerebrate cats [3–5] and also human sub-jects [6–8] on a treadmill; it revealed that the program is located in the spinal cord, and this program is now called the "central pattern generator (CPG)." We also exam-ined the functions of CPG in patients with SCI under our experimental settings. By using the training device Easy Gait Glider (Altimate Medical Inc., USA), we pro-duced passive lower limb motion in an alternating manner and recorded electro-myographic (EMG) signals in the lower limbs. Figure 3b shows the activities of each muscle that is completely paralyzed in the subject. Because we observed rhyth-mic burst from the right and left legs as observed when the limbs make stepping movements, we assumed that the CPG in this subject was activated. With the same device, we can also investigate which components of passive leg motion are critical for CPG activation. If the observed EMG activities are induced by stretch reflex in each leg, the same EMG activities are expected when only one leg is passively moved or both legs are passively moved but in a synchronized manner and not in an alternating manner. Even though the kinematic parameters of the examined leg were exactly the same under the experimental conditions, we only observed a gait-like EMG pattern in those patients who showed passive leg motion in an alternating

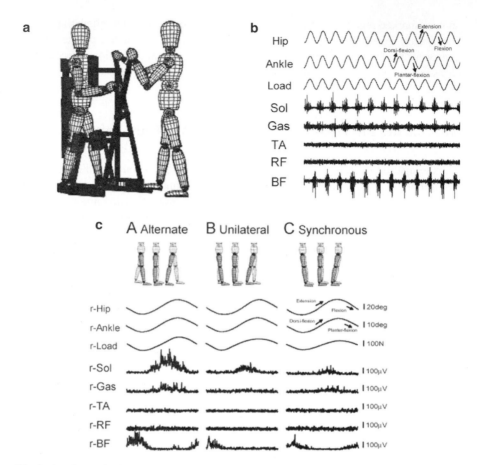

Fig. 3 An electrophysiological approach to incomplete SCI. For patients with incomplete SCI, we have shown that the activation of the central pattern generator is one of the key elements for the restoration of locomotive function. (**a**) Passive leg exercise using the Easy Stand Glider. (**b**) Phasic EMG activities in the soleus (Sol), gastrocnemius (Gas), and biceps femoris (BF) muscles during passive leg exercise in patients with complete SCI. (**c**) Alternate leg motion is necessary for the induction of gait-like EMG activities. Even though kinematic parameters are equivalent, EMG activities evoked during alternate passive leg motion are much stronger than those evoked during unilateral or synchronous leg motion

manner (Fig. 3c). These results indicate that CPG activation is specific to afferent stimuli resulting from alternate leg motion [9].

The existence of spinal CPG in individuals with and without SCI gives an idea of the kind of strategy required for rehabilitation of patients with incomplete SCI. Because CPG activation plays a pivotal role in locomotion, optimization of CPG activities will improve locomotive functions for those classified as Frankel C. In a more systematic manner, we envision a possible three-step approach, including (1) application of correct afferent input, (2) utilization of intersegmental coordination (this refers to a combination of the leg and arm swing), and (3) production of a descending command from the cortex. To develop an optimized CPG activation training protocol, electrophysiology is one of noninvasive approaches for evaluating the activities of CPG. For example, the second component of the above scheme, i.e., inter-segmental coordination, can be tested using the Easy Stand Glider. Kawashima et al. performed experiments in which patients with SCI were placed in the Easy Stand Glider while their arms were resting or were in passive or active swing, and alternative passive motion was applied to the lower limbs with the same kinematics [10]. In this experiment, they observed that along with arm swing, the subjects showed more gait-like EMG activation in their lower limbs. Interestingly, abnormal EMG activity, such as unfavorable contraction of the soleus muscle during swing phase, was reduced in some subjects when they were made to perform arm swing as well. Taken together, they concluded that the arm swing will facilitate CPG activation both by both promoting physiological EMG pattern and reducing abnormal EMG pattern.

Because passive gait training induces CPG activation as described above, it is reasonable to apply these principles for the rehabilitation of patients with incomplete SCI. For such a purpose, the recently developed training device Lokomat (Hocoma, Zurich, Switzerland) is useful. Lokomat is an exoskeleton gait assistive device, which controls the hip and knee joints of subjects on body weight-supported treadmill [11]. The concept is based on assistive gait training provided by a physiotherapist. Taking advantage of automated assistance and robotic machinery, Lokomat can provide reproducible gait kinematics with a few non-physiotherapists. Because Lokomat provides physiologically oriented gait-like kinematics to subjects, passive gait training using Lokomat is expected to induce CPG activation in the same manner, or even in a more efficient manner, as observed when using the Easy Stand Glider. Further investigation studies should focus on whether the activation of CPG during training sessions has any long-lasting effects on the locomotive function of subjects.

A Novel Approach for Evaluating Prognosis of Patients with SCI

Some novel approaches for patients with complete and incomplete SCI, including the abovementioned Lokomat training method, are being tested in the preclinical stage. For the application of these therapies, the methods of evaluating the spinal condition are also very important. In particular, it should be noted that spontaneous recovery has been observed in patients with SCI in Frankel B–C. It has been reported that on admission, patients who presented with SCI of Frankel B to C showed significant spontaneous recovery within several months to a year [12]. Therefore, it is hard to determine the efficacy of any therapeutic intervention on the basis of the functional recovery in each patient. Thus far, a neurological examination is the only means of assessing the severity of the injury; however, alternative methods of evaluating the severity of the condition are required.

For diagnosing central nervous system disorders, the use of blood and cerebrospinal fluid (CSF) samples and the measurement of specific protein levels have also been attempted. The proteins are regarded as biomarkers as they help monitor the disorder. For example, the intracellular calcium binding protein S100B has been a candidate biomarker for patients with subarachnoid hemorrhage [13]. Because the glial cells in the brain are enriched with the S100B protein, S100B is thought to be released in the blood upon damage to the cells, which leads to its increased expression in the blood. As for patients with SCI, there are not many reports on useful biomarkers for this condition. Kwon et al. measured CSF levels in 30 patients with SCI and found a certain correlation with functional severity [14]. However, it is not always feasible to obtain CSF samples from patients with acute phase SCI; therefore, it is preferable to obtain information from blood samples.

Recently, Shaw et al. reported that a certain type of neurofilament, i.e., the phosphorylated form of a high-molecular-weight neurofilament subunit NF-H (pNF-H) [15], is released into the blood after damage of the central nervous tissue and is more stable compared to conventional biomarker candidates. Therefore, the elevated concentration of pNF-H in the blood is thought to reflect axonal damage of the neural tissue. In contrast to the other biomarkers of neural injury, pNF-H can be detected after 24 h in experimental spinal cord contusion injury in rodents and peaks 3–4 days later, whereas most other biomarkers peak within 24 h. The time point at which the pNF-H level best reflects the initial severity of the trauma remains unknown. Further, pNF-H can be a useful tool for evaluating the efficacy of pharmacological intervention in patients with acute SCI because pNF-H can be detected in the blood for several days and may reflect progression of secondary injury to axons. In our recent work, we examined the pNF-H concentration in SCI rats treated with either intraperitoneal administration of minocycline or saline (control). Minocycline is known to be a neuroprotective drug and several reports have revealed its efficacy in functional recovery in an animal SCI model [16]. Under our experimental conditions, we also confirmed the effectiveness of minocycline using the end-point functional motor score of the hind limb of rats (28 days after injury) (Fig. 4b). At the same time, the level of pNF-H in the plasma shows a difference 3–4 days after injury (Fig. 4a). The minocycline-treated group tended to have a lower pNF-H level, which was in accordance with their improved motor recovery. Taken together, the pNF-H level can be used not only as a diagnostic tool for the initial severity of SCI but also as a monitoring tool after therapeutic intervention. It still needs to be investigated whether pNF-H is measurable in patients with SCI and whether it can serve as a biomarker.

Conclusion

We have discussed the possibilities of the use of the electrophysiological and molecular approaches for SCI treatment. Although a direct combination of the two paradigms is not feasible at the moment, we can select either method depending on the clinical problem that needs to be solved. Generally, the molecular approach is useful when attempting to restore or preserve neural tissue structure, i.e., the hardware of the spinal cord, whereas the electrophysiological approach can be used for modulating

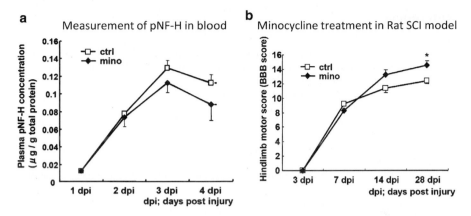

Fig. 4 A molecular approach for evaluating the severity of SCI. The phosphorylated form of high-molecular-weight neurofilament subunit NF-H (pNF-H) is a novel biomarker of central nervous system disorders. (**a**) The plasma pNF-H concentration was compared between minocycline-treated and saline-treated groups in SCI induced in rats. The reduction in the pNF-H level at 3 and 4 days after the injury in minocycline-treated groups indicate less axonal damage in this group. (**b**) The reduction in the plasma pNF-H level coincides better with functional recovery in the hind limb

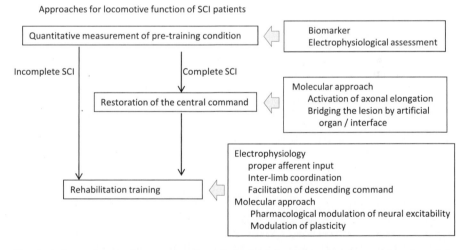

Fig. 5 A frame format of approaches for spinal cord injury. Even though a combination of the molecular and electrophysiological methods is difficult, we can use either methodology, depending on the clinical problem that needs to be solved

or evaluating use-dependent plasticity, or in other words the software of spinal neural circuits. To solve various clinical problems in SCI, the first step is to clarify the therapeutic target in each case. Further, we should prepare proper evaluation systems on the basis of the therapeutic targets, in which we can use both electrophysiological and molecular approaches (Fig. 5).

References

1. Miura T, Tanaka S, Seichi A, Arai M, Goto T, Katagiri H, Asano T, Oda H, Nakamura K (2000) Partial functional recovery of paraplegic rat by adenovirus-mediated gene delivery of constitutively active MEK1. Exp Neurol 166:115–126
2. Basso DM, Beattie MS, Bresnahan JC (1995) A sensitive and reliable locomotor rating scale for open field testing in rats. J Neurotrauma 12:1–21
3. Duysens J, Pearson KG (1980) Inhibition of flexor burst generation by loading ankle extensor muscles in walking cats. Brain Res 187:321–332
4. Grillner S (1985) Neurobiological bases of rhythmic motor acts in vertebrates. Science 228:143–149
5. Pearson KG (1995) Proprioceptive regulation of locomotion. Curr Opin Neurobiol 5:786–791
6. Dimitrijevic MR, Gerasimenko Y, Pinter MM (1998) Evidence for a spinal central pattern generator in humans. Ann N Y Acad Sci 860:360–376
7. Dietz V, Harkema SJ (2004) Locomotor activity in spinal cord-injured persons. J Appl Physiol 96:1954–1960
8. Dietz V, Müller R, Colombo G (2002) Locomotor activity in spinal man: significance of afferent input from joint and load receptors. Brain 125:2626–2634
9. Kawashima N, Nozaki D, Abe MO, Akai M, Nakazawa K (2005) Alternate leg movement amplifies locomotor-like muscle activity in spinal cord injured persons. J Neurophysiol 93:777–785
10. Kawashima N, Nozaki D, Abe MO, Nakazawa K (2008) Shaping appropriate locomotive motor output through interlimb neural pathway within spinal cord in humans. J Neurophysiol 99:2946–2955
11. Colombo G, Wirz M, Dietz V (2001) Driven gait orthosis for improvement of locomotor training in paraplegic patients. Spinal Cord 39:252–255
12. Singhal B, Mohammed A, Samuel J, Mues J, Kluger P (2008) Neurological outcome in surgically treated patients with incomplete closed traumatic cervical spinal cord injury. Spinal Cord 46:603–607
13. Moritz S, Warnat J, Bele S, Graf BM, Woertgen C (2010) The prognostic value of NSE and S100B from serum and cerebrospinal fluid in patients with spontaneous subarachnoid hemorrhage. J Neurosurg Anesthesiol 22:21–31
14. Kwon BK, Stammers AM, Belanger LM, Bernardo A, Chan D, Bishop CM, Slobogean GP, Zhang H, Umedaly H, Giffin M, Street J, Boyd MC, Paquette SJ, Fisher CG, Dvorak MF (2010) Cerebrospinal fluid inflammatory cytokines and biomarkers of injury severity in acute human spinal cord injury. J Neurotrauma 27:669–682
15. Shaw G, Yang C, Ellis R, Anderson K, Parker Mickle J, Scheff S, Pike B, Anderson DK, Howland DR (2005) Hyperphosphorylated neurofilament NF-H is a serum biomarker of axonal injury. Biochem Biophys Res Commun 336:1268–1277
16. Ueno T, Ohori Y, Ito J, Hoshikawa S, Yamamoto S, Nakamura K, Tanaka S, Akai M, Tobimatsu Y, Ogata T (2010) Hyperphosphorylated neurofilament NF-H as a biomarker of the efficacy of minocycline therapy for spinal cord injury. Spinal Cord 49:333–336. doi:10.1038/sc.2010.116

Part II
Augmenting Cognition

Prism Adaptation and the Rehabilitation of Spatial Neglect

Sophie Jacquin-Ciourtois, Jacinta O'Shea, Jacques Luauté, Laure Pisella, Alessandro Farné, Patrice Revol, Gilles Rode, and Yves Rossetti

Abstract A large proportion of right-hemisphere stroke patients exhibits spatial neglect, a neurological condition characterised by deficits for perceiving, attending, representing, and/or performing actions within their left-sided space. spatial neglect is responsible for many debilitating effects on everyday life, for poor functional recovery, and for decreased ability to benefit from treatment. Prism adaptation (PA) to a right lateral displacement of the visual field (induced by a simple target-pointing task while wearing base-left wedge prisms) is known to directionally bias visuo-motor and sensory-motor correspondences and has recently been found to improve various symptoms of neglect. For example, performance on classical pen-and-pencil visuo-motor tests could be improved for at least 2 h following adaptation. Further effects of PA have also been described for non-motor and non-visual tasks, such as for somatosensory extinction or dichotic listening, for deficits in mental imagery of geographic maps and in number bisection, and even for visuo-constructive disorders. These results

S. Jacquin-Ciourtois (✉) • J. Luauté • P. Revol • G. Rode • Y. Rossetti (✉)
Centre de recherche en Neurosciences de Lyon, Inserm U1028, CRNS UMR5092, ImpAct, 16 avenue Lépine, Bron, France
and
Université de Lyon, Université Lyon 1, Lyon, France
and
Service de Rééducation Neurologique, Plate-forme Mouvement et Handicap, Hôpital Henry Gabrielle, Hospices Civils de Lyon, Route de Vourles, 69230, St Genis Laval, France
e-mail: sophie.ciourtois@chu-lyon.fr; yves.rossetti@chu-lyon.fr

L. Pisella • A. Farné
Centre de recherche en Neurosciences de Lyon, Inserm U1028, CRNS UMR5092, ImpAct, 16 avenue Lépine, Bron, France
and
Université de Lyon, Université Lyon 1, Lyon, France

J. O'Shea
Centre for Functional Magnetic Resonance Imaging of the Brain (FMRIB), Nuffield Department of Clinical Neurosciences, University of Oxford, Oxford, UK

K. Kansaku and L.G. Cohen (eds.), *Systems Neuroscience and Rehabilitation*, DOI 10.1007/978-4-431-54008-3_6, © Springer 2011

suggest that the effects of prism adaptation can extend to unexposed sensory systems. The bottom-up approach of visuo-motor adaptation appears to interact with higher order brain functions related to multisensory integration and can have beneficial effects on sensory processing in different modalities. Lesion studies and functional imaging data point to a cerebello-cortical network in which the cerebellum is crucial for adaptation and the cortex is involved in functional gains. Prism adaptation may act not only on the ipsilesional bias characteristic of neglect and also alleviate more generally other spatial cognition deficits due to attentional bias.

Spatial Neglect, a Space-Oriented Behavioural Disorder

Spatial neglect is a fascinating neurological syndrome in which the patient fails to report, respond to, or orient toward novel and/or meaningful stimuli presented to the side opposite of the brain lesion [1, 2]. This condition is most frequently found in right-brain-damaged patients, often in association with contralesional hemiplegia, hemianesthesia, and hemianopia. Neglect thus constitutes a space-oriented behavioural disorder with an ispilesional bias, typically toward the right side. The patient spontaneously displays a tonic eye and head deviation towards the right side. This behavioural bias will be also evidenced in many clinical tests, such as in cancelling lines [3], searching for an object, or pointing to a straight-ahead position in darkness [4] (see Fig. 1). The core phenomenon of neglect is that this behavioural ipsilesional bias is associated with unawareness of contralesional space [5–7]. Neglect patients are thus unable to compensate their illness by a voluntary orientation of attention – contrasting with hemianopic patients who can orient their gaze toward the blind hemifield.

Severe and persistent spatial neglect is predominantly consecutive to lesions of the right hemisphere [7, 8]. The first damaged cortical area evidenced was the inferior parietal lobule (Brodmann areas 39 and 40) [9, 10]. Damage to other areas, such as Brodmann areas 6, 8, and 44, and to the superior temporal sulcus could also produce neglect, along with damage to sub-cortical structures and white matter fibres [11–15]. In addition to the variety and widespread nature of the lesions, many component deficits have been proposed to underlie neglect (see reviews in [16, 17]): a disorder of directing attention to the left [18–21]; an impaired representation of space, which can be in multiple frames of reference (for example, retinotopic, head centred, trunk centred) [22, 23]; and a directional motor impairment affecting the programming and initiation of contralesional eye or limb movements [24]. These proposed lateralised component deficits are not mutually exclusive, and several may coexist within the same neglect patient, having both parietal and frontal lesions [25]. More recently, some investigations have pointed some associated non-spatially lateralized deficits [16] (as non lateralized selective attention, non-spatially lateralized sustained attention, spatial working memory, spatial remapping). These mechanisms are not specific but could exacerbate severity of neglect when they are combined with lateralized components.

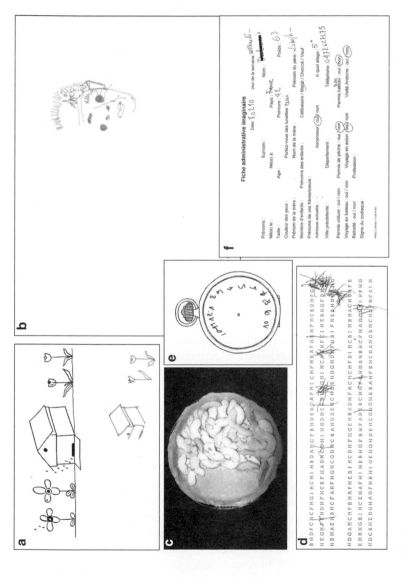

Fig. 1 Unilateral neglect. Spatial neglect is a space-oriented behaviour disorder with an ipsilesional bias, typically toward the right side. This bias may be evidenced in many clinical tests, such as (**a**) copying a drawing, where both space-based and object-based neglect can be observed; (**b**) letter cancellation, where both left neglect and revisiting of the right side can be observed; (**c**) making an apple tart in the occupational therapy unit; (**d**) spontaneous portrait of one of the author (YR) by a neglect patient who was an architect, showing the use of a limited space on the page and an object-centred neglect; (**e**) filling a clock face; (**f**) filling a fake administrative form (the name of the patient was made invisible) (color online)

Two Approaches in Neglect Rehabilitation

A Disabiliting Deficit

Spatial neglect induces many debilitating effects on everyday life and has been shown to be responsible for poor functional recovery and reduced ability to benefit from treatment of the impaired motor functions [26–31]. Although some spontaneous recovery occurs in the majority of patients after a stroke, left visuo-spatial neglect therefore remains severe in many patients and may persist chronically (29, 32, 33). The natural recovery of visuospatial neglect has been studied by Cassidy et al. [32] in 66 patients with acute right hemispheric stroke. The author showed that recovery toke place throughout the 3 month period but was greatest in the first month and that recovery from visuospatial neglect and recovery of daily living activities are likely to be closely linked or associated. Moreover the authors have shown that the recovery was greatest in the right hemispace consistent with the fact that attention remained biased rightward regardless of the absolute location of the target.

A significant correlation between improvement in neglect and function was also found by Farnè et al. [33] in a prospective study of 33 right-brain damaged patients (23 with neglect and 10 without). Patients were followed up for 3 months. The results showed that patients without neglect gain better distal motor control across sessions compared to neglect patients; visual neglect has therefore a negative impact on motor recovery and the angular gyrus (BA 39) was found to be involved both in the acute genesis of neglect and the maintenance of the neglect syndrome. The main open question is about how one can reduce the behavioural bias of neglect and, as a corollary, improve the consciousness of left peripersonal and personal spaces (for reviews, see [34, 35]). Two theoretical trends may be distinguished in the rehabilitation of neglect: a 'top-down' and a 'bottom-up' approach.

The Top-Down Approach

The first, pragmatic, clinical approach aimed at improving the perceptual and behavioural biases focused its action on the patient's awareness of the deficit, i.e., at the highest cognitive levels, including training in visual scanning, cueing, or sustained attention [36, 37]. The visual scanning training consists of correcting the ipsilesional deviation of behaviour (and gaze) by enclosing repetitive eye movement scanning exercises, in order to restore automatic scanning on the affected side. These training procedures produced substantial improvement in neglect patients with an additional generalisation of improvement to a variety of everyday living situations involving spatial exploration. This generalisation applied only when training lasted for between 4 consecutive weeks in the study of Diller and Weinberg [36] and 8 weeks in other studies [37–39]. The paradox of this approach was already underlined by Diller and Weinberg [36]: the first step in the treatment of hemi-inattention is to make the patient aware of the problem. This is particularly difficult in hemi-inattention since this failure in awareness appears to be at the heart of the patient's difficulty'. It may indeed appear paradoxical to base a reha-bilitation procedure on awareness and intention in patients with a deficit in con-sciousness. How can a sustained overt orienting to the left be obtained from individuals whose pathology is precisely to remain unable to attend to the left? These techniques have produced significant results but clearly have several limita-tions: voluntary monitoring of attention can be improved but remain restricted to a specific context and does not apply as soon as more automatic control is required. To act on higher-level cognition in such a way as to bypass the impaired conscious awareness and intention, one should find another entry route to space representa-tion systems.

The Bottom-Up Approach

This physiological approach is aimed at modifying the sensory-motor level by pas-sive sensory manipulations, visual deprivation or by visuo-motor adaptation which bypasses the central awareness deficit and directly influences the highest levels of space and action representation ([40–43]; Kerkhoff and Rossetti 2006 [125]). Numerous manifestations of neglect have been shown to be alleviated by sensory stimulation (vestibular, optokinetic, transcutaneous electrical, transcutaneous mechanical vibratory and auditory). The efficacy of repetitive optokinetic stimula-tion (OKS) with active pursuit eye movements toward the left side was assessed by Kherkhoff and colleagues in different studies. The authors have recently compared this method to conventional visual scanning training (SCT) in two groups of seven neglect patients. Each group received the same amount of repetitive OKS or conven-tional SCT. The results showed a greater effect of OKS treatment in all five patients, a generalization across all tasks. The amelioration of neglect symptoms after OKS training is associated with a pattern of activation representing a combination of areas normally involved in spatial attention plus a compensatory recruitment of left hemisphere areas [44]. These results suggest that the OKS by a bottom-up track may facilitate the generation of a more accurate egocentric space representation, by providing directional, visual motion input to this disturbed spatial representation in neglect patients.

The reversibility of various symptoms of neglect therefore suggests that a specific functional component is associated with damage to the right hemisphere. This may be explained by the fact that neglect follows damage of multimodal areas related to the orientation of spatial behaviours, and not to primary sensory or motor cortical areas. These associative areas can be activated by stimulation of various sensory modalities [45, 46] and may be organised in parallel with other central nervous system structures which receive convergent multisensory inputs thereby modulating the functional deficits.

Prism Adaptation

A Behavioural Bias Induced in Normal Subjects

In normal subjects, a behavioural bias may be experimentally induced by a simple prism adaptation procedure (reviews: [47, 48]). The relevant point for neglect rehabilitation is that after a rightward optical deviation of the visual field, subjects show a systematic leftward deviation of visuo-motor and proprioceptive responses with the adapted limb. The idea proposed by Rossetti and colleagues [49] was to use this after-effect as method to help neglect patients re-orient their behaviour towards the neglected side (see Fig. 2). This re-orientation is such that it may be produced without requiring the patient's voluntary attention, i.e., according to a bottom-up process that bypasses awareness and intentional control [50].

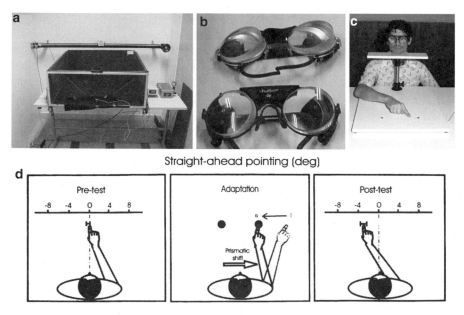

Fig. 2 Prism adaptation. (**a**) The pointing table used by Rossetti et al. in 1998 and several subsequent studies, allowing the experimenter to measure closed-loop and open-loop pointing performance in the dark, as well as the visual and the manual straight ahead. (**b**) Prismatic glasses fitted with 10 and 15° prisms. (**c**) Light version of the prism adaptation table used in several clinical studies. (**d**) Schematic description of the basic principle of prism adaptation. Healthy individuals normally can point straight ahead in the dark accurately (pre-test). During a session of several minutes of pointing to visual target while wearing the prisms, subjects progressively reduce heir initially biased performance to the right (if the optical shift is to the right). At the end of this exercise, their manual pointing is biased to the left (compensatory after-effects are measured by substracting post-tests and pre-tests) (color online)

Improvement of Visual Neglect

In the first prism rehabilitation study, Rossetti and colleagues [49] demonstrated that a short period of pointing (50 movements over 2–5 min) towards targets viewed under a 10° rightward displacement, resulted in a shift in manual straight-ahead pointing toward the left side [after the exposure the neglect patients produced an average pointing bias of just 2° rightward, i.e., showing an after-effect of about 8° (or 80% compensation for the 10° optical displacement)]. This shift of propriocep-tive representations toward the neglected side was associated with a reduction of the rightward bias observed in visuo-manual tasks, such as line cancellation [3], line bisection [51], and drawing a daisy from memory.

Following this initial study, numerous papers have subsequently been published about the effects of PA on symptoms of neglect. These main results are summarized in Table 1. In most studies, the main tests used to assess the effects of prism training required a visuo-manual response, that is, the use of the physiological systems that are directly involved in the adaptation procedure. Crucially however, some results showed that the beneficial effects of prism training are not restricted merely to visuo-motor tasks, but can also be observed for non-motor and non-visual tasks such as somatosensory and auditory extinction. The following sections will describe some of these studies.

Sensory Effects

The non-visual sensory effects of prism adaptation provide key arguments for the high generalisation of this procedure. McIntosh et al. [56] have assessed effect of prism adaptation on a spatial judgement task in a single chronic neglect patient. In this task, with no direct explicit visual component, the patient had to locate the centre of a haptically explored circle. Patient was examined in four sessions, spaced at weekly intervals, at approximately 9 months post-stroke. In each session, a neglect test battery was administered; prism adaptation (rightward optical shift to 10°) was performed at the three last sessions. Results showed not only improve-ment of symptoms of neglect at a chronic stage and but also positive results on a spatial task with no explicit visual component, already suggesting a recalibration of a high-level representation of space. These effects could reflect changes in cen-tral cognitive processes involved in the representation of space, supporting the hypothesis that a low-level sensori-motor intervention can exert a bottom-up struc-turing influence on higher levels of cognitive integration. Further studies described an improvement of tactile or proprioceptive threshold and extinction following prism adaptation (see Table 1).

The most striking observation was obtained with auditory modality, which is fully independent from the visuo-manual system involved in prism adaptation.

Table 1 Summary view of relevant papers studying the prism adaptation effects in right-brain-damaged patients with neglect

Deficiencies	
Visuo-motor tasks (bisection, cancellation, drawing, …)	[52]
	[53]
	[54]
	[55]*
	[56]*
	[57]
	[58, 59]
	[60]*
	[61]*
	[123]
	[62]*
	[63]
	[64]
	[65, 66]*
	[67]*
	[124]
	[68, 69]
	[70]*
	[71]*
	[72]*
	[73]
Visuo-verbal tasks (object or room description, reading, TOJ)	[52]
	[53]
	[55]*
	[56]*
	[74]
	[122]
	[75]
	[76]
	[62]*
	[67]*
	[77]
Oculo-motor exploration	[78]
	[74]
	[75]
	[79]*
	[80]
	[62]*
	[123]
	[63]*
SomatosensoryHaptic tasks, tactile threshold or extinction	[56]*
	[81]
	[82]*
	[62]*

(continued)

Table 1 (continued)

Deficiencies	
Auditory	[83]
Extinction, auditory attention	[71]
Representational neglect	[49, 84]
Visual and number mental imagery	[85]
Visuo-constructive disorders	[58, 59]
	[50]
Disabilities	
Manual wheel-chair driving	[86]
	[87]
Reading	[52]
	[53]
	[75]
	[67]*
Writing	[58, 59]
Daily life activities	[55]*
	[61]*
	[70]*
	[72]*
Handicap	
	No study available

*Indicates repeated sessions

Recently, Jacquin-Courtois et al. [83] have assessed prism adaptation effect on auditory extinction, an auditory deficit occurring frequently in right brain-damaged patients with neglect. This deficit, whose clinical manifestations are independent of the sensory modalities engaged in visuo-manual adaptation was examined in neglect patients before and after prism adaptation, by means of a dichotic listening task (Fig. 3).

The results demonstrated that prism adaptation can improve left auditory extinction, thus revealing transfer of benefit to a sensory modality that is orthogonal to the visual, proprioceptive and motor modalities directly implicated in the visuo-motor adaptive process. The observed benefit was specific to the detection asymmetry between the two ears and did not affect the total number of responses. This indicates a specific effect of prism adaptation on lateralized processes rather than on general arousal. The results suggest that the effects of prism adaptation can extend to unexposed sensory systems. The bottom-up approach of visuo-motor adaptation appears to interact with higher order brain functions related to multisensory integration and can have beneficial effects on sensory processing in different modalities.

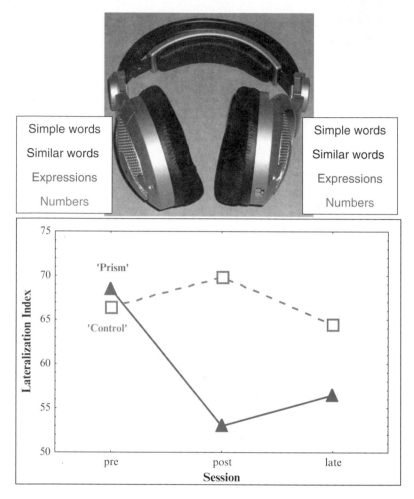

Fig. 3 Auditory effects of prism adaptation. Patients were presented simultaneously with two words and asked to repeat everything they could hear. Before prism adaptation, the two groups showed a similar number of omissions of left-sided stimuli (as reflected by the lateralisation index). After the 5 min prism adaptation exercise, only the group wearing real prisms improved and this effect lasted for at least 2 h (from [83]) (color online)

Cognitive Effects

In addition to these sensory effects, other results showed that beneficial effects of prism adaptation can also be described for both non- visual and non- motor tasks such as mental imagery of geographic maps and in mental number bisection (see Table 1). Figure 4 shows the positive effects of prism adaptation on the evocation of towns evoked by the mental visualisation of the map of France and on mental number bisection.

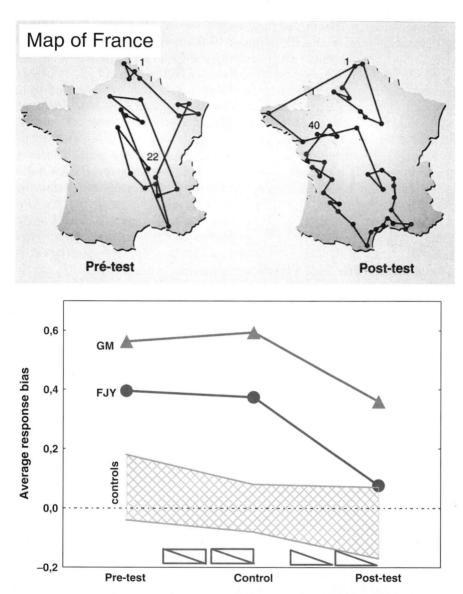

Fig. 4 The effects of prism adaptation on mental imagery. (*Top*) Towns of France named by a patient before and after prism adaptation. The patient wears a blindfold and is asked to mentally imagine the map, and then to name all towns they can see on this mental map. The experimenter plots the towns in the evoked order (from [49]). (*Bottom*) The effect of prism adaptation on mental number bisection. Subjects are orally presented with two numbers and their task is to evaluate where the central value is, without making calculation. In this example 2 patients and a group of controls have been tested before prism adaptation, following a sham prism adaptation session, and following real prism adaptation session (from [85]) (color online)

These findings suggest the recalibration of visuo-motor transformations induced by prism exposure may influence the higher-level supramodal representations associated with spatial attention. The bottom-up approach of visuo-motor adaptation appears to interact with higher order brain functions related to multisensory integration and can have beneficial effects in turn on unexposed sensory processing. Moreover effects of PA were reported in patients showing neglect dysgraphia or constructional deficits. Interestingly, this beneficial effect concerned not only the left part of the model or the text, but also the ipsilesional right part [58, 59]. This data further supports the idea that PA might improve spatial-cognition deficits in neglect as well as in pathologies such as in constructional deficits and other pathological manifestations affecting spatial and bodily representations (e.g. Complex Regional Pain Syndrome) [77, 88, 89].

Therapeutic Effects of Prism Adaptation

Chronic Versus Acute Stage Exposure

An improvement has also been obtained in patients with chronic neglect of 9 months, 5 years, and even of 19 years duration [56, 60, 90]. These clinical findings therefore suggest that low-level, automatic modifications of visuo-motor correspondence induced by prism exposure may influence visuo-spatial awareness even after a long post-stroke delay in right-brain-damaged patients. In a distinctive study, Shiraishi et al. [63] have tested seven chronic neglect patients (over 1 year from onset). Prism adaptation was performed with activity performance instead of pointing performance and the efficacy was assessed by changes in eye movements (degrees), intentional spatial bias (centre of gravity) and regional cerebral blood flow (rCBF). Prism adaptation was very originally performed about four times per week over 8 weeks. Each session (50 min) consisted into tossing rings, performing a pegboard exercise and various activities while wearing prismatic glasses. The effects of the intervention were assessed before and immediately after the intervention (immediate effects) and 1 h after the end of the first session (short-term effects). The long-term effects were also assessed by measuring the degree of eye movements at 1 and 3 days and 1, 2, 3, 4, 5, and 6 weeks after the 8-week intervention. The results show a leftward shift of eye movements and of centre of gravity compared with the base line and these improvements lasted for up to 6 weeks. Furthermore, rCBF showed a significant increase in the parietal cortex, pericallosal area of the left hemisphere. The authors conclude that long-term intervention could be useful in the chronic phase and that the use of the unaffected limb in various activities while wearing prism glasses could be important factors for understanding the effects of prism exposure.

Nys et al. [65, 66] assessed the effectiveness of repetitive prism adaptation (four consecutive sessions) in the treatment of *acute* neglect, during their stay on the stroke unit (within 4 weeks post-stroke), based on the hypothesis that the brain is more sensitive to rehabilitative treatment early after stroke. Sixteen acute stroke patients have been tested, ten receiving experimental treatment (rightward optical shift of 10°) and six placebo treatment (0° shift). Treatment and PA effect measures were administered in four daily consecutive sessions which took about 30 min each in both conditions. An immediate effect assessment (line bisection, copying task, cancellation task) and a long-term effect assessment (BIT) were performed. Results showed no apparent reduction in after effects over repeated sessions. A faster improvement was yet noted in the prism group compared to the control group during the first weeks post-stroke with respect to hemispatial performance. However, this difference was no longer observed at 1 month post-treatment. In their double blind clinical trial on 39 negelct patients, Mizuno et al. [126] found that sub-acute patients were improved by repeated sessions of prism adaptation when tested at discharge.

Taken altogether the available data suggest that although no upper limit seems to constrain the therapeutic use of prism adaptation in neglect patients, clear evidence that it can significantly improve the evolution of acute patients is still lacking.

Single Versus Repeated Exposure

The study of Rossetti and others [52] showed that improvement of neglect after a single session of adaptation was sustained over at least the 2-h follow-up period. Improvements also extended to about 1–4 days in single cases of neglect [54, 58, 59, 86], and to 1 day in a group of five neglect patients [53], showing that the effects produced by a single 5-min session of adaptation may last for much longer than any other rehabilitation method.

Using repeated sessions (including twice-daily sessions over a period of 2 weeks) in a group of seven neglect patients, and compared to an unmatched control group of six patients, Frassinetti et al. [55] demonstrated an improvement in the experimental patient's performance after PA, which was maintained over a 5-week post-treatment. This long-term improvement of neglect symptoms was found both in standard as well as in non-standard behavioural tests. Unfortunately their non-randomised control group was selected from a different hospital. Vangkilde and Habekost [72] have more recently also used the same PA regime (twice-daily sessions over a period of 2 weeks) in six patients with chronic spatial neglect and have compared their performances to a matched control group of five neglect patients receiving general cognitive rehabilitation. Assessment of neglect was performed at baseline, within a day or two after training and 5 weeks later, including clinical testing (cancellation and copying), visual search task with eye movement recording and a questionnaire for behavioural observations in daily life. Results showed significant amelioration of neglect symptoms after the training program, at few days following training as well at the 5-week follow-up. In particular, a persistent positive effect on everyday activities was noted.

As described above, Shiraishi et al. [63] observed a long lasting improvement after a long-term intervention in a chronic neglect patients group. Using ten daily sessions over a period of 2 weeks, Serino et al. [62] also reported improvement of personal and extrapersonal neglect in a group of 21 right brain damaged patients without control group. Using repeated sessions [18 sessions of PA training (two per week over 9 weeks)], Humphreys and co-workers [60] reported finding a long lasting beneficial effect in one chronic patient, which was maintained up to a year following the PA training. Serino et al. [67] conducted a study to investigate the effectiveness on neglect recovery of a 2-week treatment (ten daily sessions) based on prism adaptation (PA) (ten patients) in comparison to an analogous visuomotor training performed without prisms, i.e., neutral pointing (NP) (ten patients). After the end of NP treatment, the patients in the NP group were also submitted to PA treatment. Neglect was assessed with the BIT battery (conventional and behavioral scales) before and after each treatment and 1 month after the end of the PA treatment. Visuospatial abilities improved after both PA and NP treatment, but the improvement was significantly higher in the patients in the PA group than in the patients in the NP group. Moreover, when the patients in the NP group were submitted to PA, they further improved up to the level reached by patients in the PA group. Long-lasting beneficial effects of repetitive PA were confirmed 1 month from the end of treatment. The leftward recalibration induced by PA is effective to obtain neglect improvement, although visuomotor training based on pointing might partially improve neglect symptoms.

Negative Studies

Nevertheless negative results were also reported showing a reduction of behavioural ipsilesional bias without improvement of contralesional space unawareness in tasks such as size underestimation, judgement of vertically arranged pairs of chimeric faces or free visual exploration task [74, 78, 80]. More recently, Striemer and Danckert [73] have examined the effect of PA on perceptual and motor performances using the bisection and landmark tasks in three neglect patients and a group of controls. Results showed that for neglect patients PA reduced rightward biases in bisection, but had no effect on leftward perceptual biases on the landmark task, suggesting also dissociation between perceptual and motor influences of PA in neglect patients. Pattern of PA effect in young healthy controls seems to indicate an influence on both-perceptual and motor- levels. Additional results in control subjects have been recently shown by Nijboer et al. [91] by use of saccadic eye movements to measure the effects of a left-shifting PA on spatial attention. Performance on the antisaccade task (saccade latencies, number of erroneous eye movements) before and after PA has been compared. Influence of PA on visual perception has also been investigated using a landmark task. Results indicated no effect on saccades parameters but a perceptual bias on landmark task, suggesting a differential influence on visual attention and visual perception in healthy subjects. The discrepancy between the results of studies in healthy participants and neglect patients is informative about possible underlying mechanisms, effects of PA not simply resulting in a stronger attentional focus in one visual field. Eramudugolla et al. [71] have also assessed effects of PA on attentional parameters, in neglect patients. Usual PA protocol was used and all 12 patients showed significant visuo-motor after-effects (cancellation task). No changes in their spatial bias in exogenous attention to either visual or auditory stimuli were however found, with variable individual performances suggesting implication of individual factors.

Nys et al. [65, 66] assessed in a single case patient at a chronic stage (11 months post-stroke) the effects of 4-day-in-a-row prism adaptation on neglect severity, but also on perseveration severity observed in the ipsilesional field (repetitive fixations, ipsilesional revisitings on a cancellation task or exaggeration in drawings on the ipsilesional side). The results showed a decrease in neglect severity but an increase in perseveration severity, suggesting that perseverations and neglect could be dissociated. Interestingly, the localisation of perseverative responses was gradually moved from right to left after prism adaptation, pointing out a shift of the predominant occurrence of perseverations from ipsi- to contralesional space.

Turton et al. [70] have compared two groups of neglect patients who received ten prism adaptation or sham treatments in addition to the usual therapy for neglect (one daily session, 2 weeks). No difference was observed 4 days after this treatment. It is likely that the prisms used in this study (ten dioptre prisms that shifted the field of view by less than 6° to the right) did not shift vision by a sufficient amount, as previous studies used optical shifts ranging from 10° to 15°.

In a recent study, we have also failed to show significant improvement of neglect in a trial in which we used only a light treatment regime. Prism adaptation was used weekly over 1 month, and no benefit was visible in the prism treated group after a 6 month follow-up. Altogether the above studies show that a sufficient amount of prismatic shift and after-effects are needed to produce a significant improvement of neglect, and that repeated treatment should follow a rhythm of at least a daily adaptation session.

Neural Basis of Prism Adaptation and Hypothesis

The last question is whether PA favours the spontaneous recovery of neglect or facilitates the occurrence of selective compensation mechanisms. This question refers either to the cerebral plasticity naturally evoked after the cerebral damage, or to the cerebral plasticity specifically activated by the visuo-motor adaptation task. The fact that immediate effects can be produced, and even in chronic patients, suggests that PA does not simply enhance spontaneous recovery and that specific mechanisms are at work. There has been quite some controversy in the literature concerning the neural structures involved in PA. On the one hand, neuropsychological evidence historically suggested that only cerebellar patients were impaired in PA (e.g., [92], for review, see [47]). On the other hand, imaging data suggested that the human posterior parietal cortex contralateral to the adapted arm is the only area activated during prism exposure [93].

Pisella et al. [94] established that a bilateral lesion of the superior parietal lobule, although frequently leading to an impairment of visuo-manual guidance (optic ataxia), is not crucially involved in visuo-manual PA. The clinical effect of PA on visual neglect also precludes the possibility that the inferior parietal lobule, at least in the right hemisphere, might be crucial for adaptation to rightward prisms. A simple model was therefore proposed in which the cerebellum and the posterior parietal cortex are respectively specialised for the adaptive and strategic components of PA [95, 96]. In a patient with a cerebellar lesion (including the superior part of the dentate nucleus and the anterior lobe of the left cerebellar hemisphere), Pisella and colleagues [97] found that adaptation was limited to a rightward (not leftward) prism deviation, independently of the hand used during exposure. This observation confirmed the crucial involvement of the cerebellum in PA, and led Pisella and her collaborators to propose a lateralized model for PA and its beneficial effect on spatial cognition. The pattern of impairments in this patient suggested a visual lateralization within the cerebellum, with the involvement of the cerebellar hemisphere ipsilateral to the prismatic deviation in the processing of visual errors, in addition to the well-known motor lateralization that primarily involves the cerebellar hemisphere contralateral to the hand in the modification of visuo-motor correspondences [98]. Since connections between the cerebellum and the cerebral cortex are crossed [99], this makes a consistent cerebro-cerebellar lateralised network for the computation and integration of directional visual error in PA. The implication of such a lateralised cerebello-cerebral network in the functional anatomy of the therapeutic effects of PA on neglect has been recently confirmed by a neuroimaging study in neglect patients showing that rCBF in the right cerebellar hemisphere and the right dentate nucleus covaried significantly with improvement in neglect (assessed by the Behavioural Inattention Test). Activation of the left temporal cortex also appeared to covary positively with the improvement in left spatial neglect [100]. Moreover the fact that prism adaptation after-effects generalize across such a wide range of functions suggests that adaptation may modify a common level of spatial representation important for multisensory integration [52]. That adaptation can also improve higher-order aspects of spatial cognition (e.g. mental imagery, constructional deficits, [49]), both by reducing lateralized bias and enlarging the represented space, further suggests that prism adaptation might be used to treat not only neglect, but a range of spatial cognition disorders and visuospatial dysfunctions [50, 58, 59]. The question arises about the possible neural substrates of this higher order representation. Our current model of prism adaptation proposes that prism-induced cerebellar effects interact with contralateral posterior parietal cortex [96]. The implication of such a lateralized cerebello-cerebral network has been recently confirmed by a neuroimaging study in neglect patients [100]. More recently, Danckert et al. [101] have used fMRI paradigm to explore effects of prisms on visuomanual pointing in eight normal subjects. The results showed a modulation of activity in a network of brain regions when subjects pointed toward targets viewed through a wedge prism. This network, including primary motor cortex, anterior intraparietal region, anterior cingulated cortex and medial cerebellum, showed modulation in earlier pointing trials, suggesting its implication in recalibrating visuomotor commands. Luauté et al. [102] have also used fMRI to study dynamic changes in brain activity during both early and prolonged exposure to visual prisms in normals subjects. The results have reinforced the hypothesis of therapeutic effects by interacting with intact cortical areas [102]. Identification of the neural networks underlying the different components of prism adaptation and their dynamical time course provide new insights on the mechanisms by which visuomotor plasticity may interact with spatial cognition. Anterior intraparietal sulcus seems to be implied at the earliest phase of prism exposure (corresponding to the error detection step), whereas parieto-occipital sulcus was implicated in error correction. Cerebellum activity showed progressive increases during prism exposure, in accordance with a key role for spatial realignment, and could suggest that the cerebellum might promote neural changes in superior temporal cortex, which was selectively activated during the later phase of prism exposure and could mediate the effects of prism adaptation on cognitive spatial representations. Chapman et al. [103] have focalized on later stage of adaptation, when spatial realignment is predicted to occur. fMRI has been used in healthy adults performing pointing movements during leftward prism adaptation to quantify the distinctive patterns of parieto-cerebellar activity according the distinct adaptation phases: both cerebellum and inferior parietal lobe seem to be implicated not only during initial error correction phase but also in later spatial realignment phase. According to our model of prism adaptation [96], one may speculate that this late parietal activation resulted from a bottom-up action of the cerebellum on cortical structures which may explain the therapeutic effects of prism adaptation.

Another proposal is that adaptation acts through plastic modification of the integration of proprioceptive and visual information, which would be particularly beneficial in neglect patients, whose symptoms result in part from an impaired visual-motor mapping of space [104]. One could speculate that PA also induces an enlargement of this visual-motor mapping of space, not only on the left side, but also on the right side, as suggested by the improvement of constructional apraxia and spatial dysgraphia following PA [50]. Recent findings mainly point to the need for appropriately applying prism exposure conditions and quantification [105], for evaluating the role played by the type of PA (strategic vs. realignment [75, 79]), as well as the sufficient amount of adaptation (as measured in terms of after-effect) required to produce consistent neglect improvement [106].

More recently, Bultitude et al. [77] have suggested that adaptation to rightward-shifting prisms could improve neglect symptoms by alleviating the local processing bias classically induced by right temporo-parietal lesion. Five patients with right temporal-parietal junction lesions were asked to identify the global or local levels of hierarchical figures before and after visuomotor adaptation to rightward-shifting prisms. Prior to prism adaptation the patients had difficulty ignoring the local elements when identifying the global component. Following prism adaptation, however, this pattern was reversed, with greater global interference during local level identification. This result suggests that prism adaptation may improve non-spatially-lateralized deficits that contribute to the neglect syndrome. This non-lateralized improvement may potentiate the other lateralized effects and result in spreading attention and exploration over a wider range of space.

Perspectives for Rehabilitation of Neglect

Systematic investigations are still needed to determine both the optimum prism strength, frequency of treatment sessions and adaptation parameters. The recent clinical trial of Mizuno et al. [126] very interestingly combined the rigour of a well-designed clinical trial and the pragmatism of clinical approaches by testing patients at discharge instead of following a fixed delay. Importantly they showed a practical improvement on the Functional Independecy Measure (FIM) in their prism group.

One other prospective is to associate PA to others methods such as sensory stimulation in order to produce additional effects on the ipsilesional behavioural bias. Long-lasting effects on neglect and disability were thus reported. For example Schindler et al. [107] have evaluated the effects of differential treatment of visual exploration training alone or in combination with neck muscle vibration in a cross-over study of two matched groups of 10 patients with neglect; the results showed superior effects of combination treatment with a concomitant improvement in activities of daily living persisting 2 months later. Similar results have been reported after rehabilitation involving visual scanning training and trunk rotation [108] or neck muscle vibration [107] or functional electrical stimulation of the left hand [109]. More recently, Saevarsson et al. [69] have explored potential additive benefits using combination of neck vibration (NV) and prism adaptation (PA), at a chronic stage. Both experimental groups received NV for 20 min, while the second group received simultaneous PA. Results indicated for both groups an improvement of visual search performance, with additional clear improvements on visual search paper and pencil neglect tests only for the PA group. These results suggest the interest to associate two different tracks in rehabilitation of neglect in order to obtain a reduction of incapacity consecutive to neglect.

Another suggestion could be to associate the PA to a method (or treatment) acting on non-spatially lateralised component deficits. Indeed these deficits may also contribute to neglect: impairments in sustained attention [110], selective attention at central fixation [111], or in both visual fields deficit [112], a bias to local features in the visual scene [113], as well as a deficit in spatial working memory [114, 115] or in spatial remapping [104]. None of these deficits has been considered to be specific to neglect. However, such non-spatially lateralised deficits could exacerbate any directional deficit and have a significant impact on the neglect syndrome, reducing the potential for recovery [16, 116].

Recently an improvement of chronic neglect was reported after administration of guanfacine, a noradrenergic agonist which enhance the ability to maintain attention when exploring space. Preliminary findings underline the interest of neuropsychopharmacological approach in association with training method in neglect rehabilitation [117]. Results show improvement in terms of leftward spatial exploration by acting at an attentional level via dorsolateral prefrontal cortex.

The last perspective is to associate PA to transcranial stimulation. Indeed in the more recent years, cerebral trans-cranial stimulation techniques have been used to test the theorical proposal that neglect occurs because a unilateral stroke disrupts the normal balance of neural activity between the two hemispheres. This kind of approach seems to be promising in terms of therapeutic possibilities. Use of TMS has recently allowed researchers to confirm this empirical hypothesis ([118, 119]; review in [120]). Interestingly, a relative 'pathological' hyperexcitability of left parietal cortex (not directly damaged) caused by less competitive impact of right damaged parietal cortex has been observed and correlated to severity of neglect symptoms [121]. In a therapeutic perspective, transient improvement of neglect has been shown after left hemisphere stimulation by TMS. These results have not only clear implications in terms of clinical neurological rehabilitation but also better understanding of neural networks and mechanisms supporting therapeutic effects.

To summarize the ultimate aim is be to associate PA with a method relying on a different neural network in order to cumulate effects on the sensorimotor, cognitive as well as fine functional levels. The future challenge for rehabilitation of neglect will be to establish a tailored method taking into account the undamaged brain regions which could be activated by specific training techniques so as to favour the recovery of the patients deficits and reduce their subsequent handicap.

References

1. Brain WR (1941) Visual disorientation with special reference to lesions of the right cerebral hemisphere. Brain 64:244–271
2. Heilman KM, Watson RT, Valenstein E (1985) Neglect and related disorders. In: Heilman KM, Valenstein E (eds) Clinical neuropsychology. Oxford University Press, New York, pp 243–293
3. Albert ML (1973) A simple test of neglect. Neurology 23:658–664
4. Jeannerod M, Biguer B (1987) The directional coding of reaching movements. A visuomotor conception of spatial neglect. In: Jeannerod M (ed) Neurophysiological and neuropsychological aspects of neglect. Elsevier Science, Amsterdam, pp 87–113
5. Bisiach E (1999) Unilateral neglect and related disorders. In: Denes F, Pizzamiglio L (eds) Handbook of clinical and experimental neuropsychology. Psychology Press, Hove
6. Kerkhoff G (2001) Spatial hemineglect in humans. Prog Neurobiol 63:1–27
7. Halligan PW, Fink GR, Marshall JC, Vallar G (2003) Spatial cognition: evidence from visual neglect. Trends Cogn Sci 7:125–133
8. Vallar G (2001) Extrapersonal visual unilateral spatial neglect and its neuroanatomy. Neuroimage 14:552–558
9. Hécaen H, Penfield W, Bertrand C, Malmo R (1956) The syndrome of apractognosia due to lesions of the minor cerebral hemisphere. Arch Neurol Psychiatry 57:400–434
10. Heilman KM, Bowers D, Valenstein E, Watson RT (1983) Localization of lesion in neglect. In: Kertesz A (ed) Localization in neuropsychology. Academic, New York, pp 471–492
11. Karnath HO, Ferber S, Himmelbach M (2001) Spatial awareness is a function of the temporal not the posterior parietal lobe. Nature 411:950–953
12. Karnath HO, Himmelbach M, Rorden C (2002) The subcortical anatomy of human spatial neglect: putamen, caudate nucleus and pulvinar. Brain 125:350–360
13. Mort D, Malhotra P, Mannan S, Rorden C, Pambakian A, Kennard C, Husain M (2003) The anatomy of visual neglect. Brain 126:1986–1997
14. Doricchi F, Tomaiuolo F (2003) The anatomy of neglect without hemianopia: a key role for parietal-frontal disconnection? Neuroreport 14:2239–2243
15. Thiebaut de Schotten M, Urbanski M, Duffau H, Volle E, Lévy R, Dubois B, Bartolomeo P (2005) Direct evidence for a parietal-frontal pathway subserving spatial awareness in humans. Science 309:2226–2228

16. Husain M, Rorden C (2003) Non-spatially lateralized mechanisms in hemispatial neglect. Nat Neurosci 4:26–36
17. Parton A, Malhotra P, Husain M (2004) Hemispatial neglect. J Neurol Neurosurg Psychiatry 75:13–21
18. Kinsbourne M (1993) Orientational bias model of unilateral neglect: evidence from attentional gradients with hemispace. In: Robertson IH, Marshall JC (eds) Unilateral neglect: clinical and experimental studies. Erlbaum, Hillstale, pp 63–86
19. Posner MI, Walker JA, Friedrich FJ, Rafal RD (1984) Effects of parietal injury on covert orienting of attention. J Neurosci 4:1863–1874
20. Gainotti G, D'Erme P, Bartolomeo P (1991) Early orientation of attention toward the half space ipsilateral to the lesion in patients with unilateral brain damage. J Neurol Neurosurg Psychiatry 54:1082–1089
21. Smania N, Martini MC, Gambina G, Tomelleri G, Palamara A, Natale E, Marzi CA (1998) The spatial distribution of visual attention in hemineglect and extinction patients. Brain 121:1759–1770
22. Bisiach E, Berti A (1987) Dyschiria. An attempt at its systemic explanation. In: Jeannerod M (ed) Neurophysiological and neuropsychological aspects of spatial neglect. North Holland, Amsterdam, pp 183–201
23. Karnath HO (1997) Spatial orientation and the representation of space with parietal lobe lesions. Philos Trans R Soc Lond B 352:1411–1419
24. Mattingley JB, Bradshaw JL, Phillips JG (1992) Impairments of movement initiation and execution in unilateral neglect. Directional hypokinesia and bradykinesia. Brain 115:1849–1874
25. Husain M, Mattingley JB, Rorden C, Kennard C, Driver J (2000) Distinguishing sensory and motor biases in parietal and frontal neglect. Brain 123:1643–1659
26. Held JP, Pierrot-Deseilligny E, Bussel B, Perrigot M, Malier M (1975) Devenir des hémiplégies vasculaires par atteinte sylvienne en fonction du côté de la lésion. Ann Réadapt Méd Phys 4:592–604
27. Denes G, Semenza C, Stoppa E, Lis A (1982) Unilateral spatial neglect and recovery from hemiplegia: a follow-up study. Brain 105:543–552
28. Fullerton KJ, McSherry D, Stout RW (1986) Albert's test: a neglected test of perceptual neglect. Lancet 327:430–432
29. Katz N, Hartman-Macir A, Ring H, Soroker N (1999) Functional disability and rehabilitation outcome in right hemisphere damaged patients with and without unilateral spatial neglect. Arch Phys Med Rehabil 80:379–384
30. Jehkonen M, Ahonen JP, Dastidar P, Koivisto AM, Laippala P, Vikki J, Molnar G (2000) Visual neglect as a predictor of functional outcome one year after stroke. Acta Neurol Scand 101:195–201
31. Jehkonen M, Laihosalo M, Kettunen J (2006) Anosognosia after stroke: assessment, occurrence, subtypes and impact on functional outcome reviewed. Acta Neurol Scand 114:293–306
32. Cassidy TP, Lewis S, Gray CS (1998) Recovery from visuosptial neglect in stroke patients. J Neurol Neurosurg Psychiatry 64:555–557
33. Farnè A, Buxbaum LJ, Ferraro M, Frassinetti F, Whyte J, Veramonti T, Angeli V, Coslett HB, Ladavas E (2004) Patterns of spontaneous recovery of neglect and associated disorders in acute right brain-damaged paptients. J Neurol Neurosurg Psychiatry 75:1401–1410
34. Luauté J, Halligan P, Rode G, Jacquin-Courtois S, Boisson D (2006) Prism adaptation first among equals in alleviating left neglect. A review. Restor Neurol Neurosci 24:409–418
35. Luauté J, Halligan P, Rossetti Y, Rode G, Boisson D (2006) Visuo-spatial neglect: a systematic review of current interventions and their effectiveness. Neurosci Biobehav Rev 30:961–982
36. Diller L, Weinberg J (1977) Hemi-inattention in rehabilitation: the evolution of a rational remediation program. Adv Neurol 18:63–82
37. Pizzamiglio L, Antonucci G, Judica A, Montenero P, Razzano C, Zoccolotti P (1992) Cognitive rehabilitation of the hemineglect disorder in chronic patients with unilateral right brain damage. J Clin Exp Neuropsychol 14:901–923

38. Antonucci G, Guariglia C, Judica A, Magnotti L, Paolucci S, Pizzamiglio L, Zoccolotti P (1995) Effectiveness of neglect rehabilitation in a randomized group study. J Clin Exp Neuropsychol 17:383–389
39. Paolucci S, Antonucci G, Guariglia C, Magnotti L, Pizzamiglio L, Zoccolotti P (1996) Facilitatory effect of neglect rehabilitation on the recovery of left hemiplegic stroke patients: a cross-over study. J Neurol 243:308–314
40. Rubens AB (1985) Caloric stimulation and unilateral visual neglect. Neurology 35:1019–1024
41. Vallar G, Guariglia C, Rusconi ML (1997) Modulation of the neglect syndrome by sensory stimulation. In: Parietal lobe contributions to orientation in 3D space. Springer, Heidelberg, pp 555–578
42. Rossetti Y, Rode G (2002) Reducing spatial neglect by visual and other sensory manipulations: non-cognitive (physiological) routes to the rehabilitation of a cognitive disorder. In: Karnath HO, Milner AD, Vallar G (eds) The cognitive and neural bases of spatial neglect. Oxford University Press, New York, pp 375–396
43. Kerkhoff G (2003) Modulation and rehabilitation of spatial neglect by sensory stimulation. Prog Brain Res 142:257–271
44. Thimm M, Fink GR, Küst J, Karbe H, Willmes K, Sturm W (2009) Recovery from hemineglect: differential neurobiological effects of optokinetic stimulation and alertness training. Cortex 45:850–862
45. Bottini G, Sterzi R, Paulesu E, Vallar G, Cappa SF, Erminio F, Passingham RE, Frith CD, Frackowiak RS (1994) Identification of the central vestibular projections in man: a positron emission tomography activation study. Exp Brain Res 99:164–169
46. Bottini G, Karnath HO, Vallar G, Sterzi R, Frith CD, Frackowiak RS, Paulesu E (2001) Cerebral representations for egocentric space: functional-anatomical evidence from caloric vestibular stimulation and neck vibration. Brain 124:1182–1196
47. Jeannerod M, Rossetti Y (1993) Visuomotor coordination as a dissociable visual function: experimental and clinical evidence. In: Kennard CC (ed) Visual perceptual defect. I.P.R. Baillere Tindall Ltd, Baillere's Clinical Neurology, London, pp 439–460
48. Redding GM, Rossetti Y, Wallace B (2005) Applications of prism adaptation: a tutorial in theory and method. Neurosci Biobehav Rev 29:431–444
49. Rode G, Rossetti Y, Li L, Boisson D (1998) The effect of prism adaptation on neglect for visual imagery. Behav Neurol 11:251–258
50. Rode G, Revol P, Rossetti Y, Boisson D, Bartolomeo P (2007) Looking while imagining. The influence of visual input on representational neglect. Neurology 68:432–437
51. Schenkenberg T, Bradford DC, Ajax ET (1980) Line bisection with neurologic impairment. Neurology 30:509–517
52. Rossetti Y, Rode G, Pisella L, Farnè A, Li L, Boisson D, Perenin MT (1998) Prism adaptation to a rightward optical deviation rehabilitates left hemispatial neglect. Nature 395:166–169
53. Farnè A, Rossetti Y, Toniolo S, Ladavas E (2002) Ameliorating neglect with prism adaptation: visuo-manual and visuo-verbal measures. Neuropsychologia 40:718–729
54. Pisella L, Rode G, Farnè A, Boisson D, Rossetti Y (2002) Dissociated long lasting improvements of straight-ahead pointing and line bisection tasks in two unilateral neglect patients. Neuropsychologia 40:327–334
55. Frassinetti F, Angeli V, Meneghello F, Avanzi S, Ladavas E (2002) Long-lasting amelioration of visuospatial neglect by prism adaptation. Brain 125:608–623
56. McIntosh RM, Rossetti Y, Milner AD (2002) Prism adaptation improves chronic visual and haptic neglect. Cortex 38:309–320
57. Morris AP, Kritikos A, Berberovic N, Pisella L, Chambers CD, Mattingley J (2004) Prism adaptation and spatial attention: a study of visual search in normals and patients with unilateral neglect. Cortex 40:703–721
58. Rode G, Klos T, Courtois-Jacquin S, Rossetti Y (2006) Neglect and prism adaptation. A new therapeutic tool for saptial cognition disorders. Restor Neurol Neurosci 24:347–356
59. Rode G, Pisella L, Marsal L, Mercier S, Rossetti Y, Boisson D (2006) Prism adaptation improves spatial dysgraphia following right brain damage. Neuropsychologia 44:2487–2493

60. Humphreys GW, Watelet A, Riddoch MJ (2006) Long-term effects of prism adaptation in chronic visual neglect: a single case study. Cogn Neuropsychol 23:463–478
61. Keane S, Turner C, Sherrington C, Beard JR (2006) Use of Fresnel prism glasses to treat stroke patients with hemispatial neglect. Arch Phys Med Rehabil 87:1668–1672
62. Serino A, Bonifazi S, Pierfederici L, Ladavas E (2007) Neglect treatment by prism adaptation: what recovers and for how long. Neuropsychol Rehabil 17:657–687
63. Shiraishi H, Yamakawa Y, Itou A, Muraki T, Asada T (2008) Long-term effects of prism adaptation on chronic neglect after stroke. NeuroRehabilitation 23:137–151
64. Sarri M, Greenwood R, Kalra L, Husain M, Driver J (2008) Prism adaptation aftereffects in stroke patients with spatial neglect: Pathological effects on subjective straight ahead but not visual open-loop pointing. Neuropsychologia 46:1069–1080
65. Nys GM, Seurinck R, Dijkerman HC (2008) Prism adaptation moves neglect-related perseveration to contralesional space. Cogn Behav Neurol 21:249–253
66. Nys GMS, de Haan EHF, Kunneman A, de Kort PLM, Dijkerman HC (2008) Acute neglect rehabilitationusing repetitive prism adaptation: a randomized placebo-controlled trial. Restor Neurol Neurosci 26:1–12
67. Serino A, Barbiani M, Rinaldesi ML, Ladavas E (2009) Effectivenes of prism adaptation in neglect rehabilitation. A controlled trial study. Stroke 40:1392–1398
68. Saevarsson S, Kristjánsson A, Hildebrandt H, Halsband U (2009) Prism adaptation improves visual search in hemispatial neglect. Neuropsychologia 47:717–725
69. Saevarsson S, Kristjansson A, Halsband U (2010) Strength in numbers: combining neck vibration and prism adaptation produces additive therapeutic effects in unilateral neglect. Neuropsychol Rehabil 20:704–724
70. Turton AJ, O'Leary K, Gabb J, Woodward R, Gilchrist ID (2010) A single blinded randomised controlled pilot trial of prism adaptation for improving self-care in stroke patients with neglect. Neuropsychol Rehabil 20:180–196
71. Eramudugolla R, Boyce A, Irvine DR, Mattingley JB (2010) Effects of prismatic adaptation on spatial gradients in unilateral neglect: a comparison of visual and auditory target detection with central attentional load. Neuropsychologia 48:2681–2692
72. Vangkilde S, Habekost T (2010) Finding Wally: prism adaptation improves visual search in chronic neglect. Neuropsychologia 48:1994–2004
73. Striemer CL, Danckert J (2010) Dissociating perceptual and motor effects of prism adaptation in neglect. Neuroreport 21:436–441
74. Dijkerman HC, McIntosh RD, Rossetti Y, Tilikete C, Roberts RC, Milner AD (2003) Ocular scanning and perceptual size distortion in hemispatial neglect: effects of prism adaptation and sequential stimulus presentation. Exp Brain Res 153:220–230
75. Angeli V, Benassi MG, Ladavas E (2004) Recovery of oculo-motor bias in neglect patients after prism adaptation. Neuropsychologia 42:1223–1234
76. Sarri M, Kalra L, Greenwood R, Driver J (2006) Prism adaptation changes perceptual awareness for chimeric visual objects but not for chimeric faces in spatial neglect after right-hemisphere stroke. Neurocase 12:127–135
77. Bultitude JH, Rafal RD, List A (2009) Prism adaptation reverses the local processing bias in patients with right temporo-parietal junction lesions. Brain 132:1669–1677
78. Ferber S, Danckert J, Joanisse M, Goltz HC, Goodale MA (2003) Eye movements tell only half the story. Neurology 60:1826–1829
79. Serino A, Angeli V, Frassinetti F, Ladavas E (2006) Mechanisms underlying neglect recovery after prism adaptation. Neuropsychologia 44:1068–1078
80. Datié AM, Paysant J, Destainville S, Sagez A, Beis JM, André JM (2006) Eye movements and visuoverbal descriptions exhibit heterogeneous and dissociated patterns before and after prismatic adaptation in unilateral spatial neglect. Eur J Neurol 13:772–779
81. Maravita A, McNeil J, Malhotra P, Greenwood R, Husain M, Driver J (2003) Prism adaptation can improve contralesional tactile perception in neglect. Neurology 60:1829–1831
82. Dijkerman HC, Webeling M, Walter JM, Groet E, van Zandvoort MJ (2004) A long-lasting improvementof somatosensory function after prism adaptation, a case study. Neuropsychologia 42:1697–1702

83. Jacquin-Courtois S, Rode G, Pavani F, O'Shea J, Giard MH, Boisson D, Rossetti Y (2010) Effect of prism adaptation on left dichotic listening deficit in neglect patients: glasses to hear better? Brain 133:895–908
84. Rode G, Rossetti Y, Boisson D (2001) Prism adaptation improves representational neglect. Neuropsychologia 39:1250–1254
85. Rossetti Y, Jacquin-Courtois S, Rode G, Ota H, Michel C, Boisson D (2004) Does action make the link between number and space representation? Visuo-manual adaptation improves number bisection in unilateral neglect. Psychol Sci 15:426–430
86. Jacquin-Courtois S, Rode G, Boisson D, Rossetti Y (2008) Wheel-chair driving improvement following visuo-manual prism adaptation. Cortex 44:90–96
87. Watanabe S, Amimoto K (2010) Generalization of prism adaptation for whellchair driving task in patients with unilateral spatial neglect. Arch Phys Med Rehabil 91:443–447
88. Sumitani M, Shibata M, Yagisawa M, Mashimo T, Miyauchi S (2006) Prism adaptation to optical deviation alleviates complex regional pain syndrome: longitudinal single case study. Neurorehabil Neural Repair 20:141–142
89. Sumitani M, Rossetti Y, Shibata M, Matsuda Y, Sakaue G, Inoue T, Mashimo T, Miyauchi S (2007) Prism adaptation to optical deviation alleviates pathological pain. Neurology 68:128–133
90. Rode G, Pisella L, Rossetti Y, Farnè A, Boisson D (2003) Bottom-up transfer of sensory-motor plasticity to recovery of spatial cognition: visuomotor adaptation and spatial neglect. Prog Brain Res 142:273–287
91. Nijboer T, Vree A, Dijkerman C, Van der Stigchel S (2010) Prism adaptation influences perception but not attention: evidence from antisaccades. Neuroreport 21:386–389
92. Weiner MJ, Hallett M, Funkenstein HH (1983) Adaptation to lateral displacement of vision in patients with lesions of the central nervous system. Neurology 33:766–772
93. Clower DM, Hoffman JM, Votaw JR, Fabert TL, Woods R, Alexander GE (1996) Role of posterior parietal cortex in the recalibration of visually guide reaching. Nature 383:618–621
94. Pisella L, Michel C, Grea H, Tilikete C, Vighetto A, Rossetti Y (2004) Preserved prism adaptation in bilateral optic ataxia: strategic versus adaptive reaction to prisms. Exp Brain Res 156:399–408
95. Rossetti Y, Pisella L, Colent C (2000) A cerebellar therapy for a parietal deficit? (abstract). In: Weiss PHH (ed) Action and visuo-spatial attention, neurobiological bases and disorders. Life Sciences, Reihe Lebenswissenschaften, Forschungszentrum Jülich GmbH, Germany, p 21
96. Pisella L, Rode G, Farnè A, Tilikete C, Rossetti Y (2006) Prism adaptation in the rehabilitation of patients with visuo-spatial cognitive disorders. Curr Opin Neurol 19:534–542
97. Pisella L, Rossetti Y, Michel C, Rode G, Boisson D, Pélisson D, Tilikete C (2005) Ipsidirectional impairment of prism adaptation after unilateral lesion of anterior cerebellum. Neurology 65:150–152
98. Martin TA, Keating JG, Goodkin HP, Bastian AJ, Thatch WT (1996) Throwing while looking through prisms, I Focal olivocerebellar lesions impair adaptation. Brain 119:1183–1198
99. Schmahmann JD (1998) Dysmetria of thought: clinical consequences of cerebellar dysfunction on cognition and affect. Trends Cogn Sci 2:362–371
100. Luauté J, Michel C, Rode G, Pisella L, Jacquin-Courtois S, Costes N, Cotton F, le Bars D, Boisson D, Halligan P, Rossetti Y (2006) Functional anatomy of the therapeutic effects of prism adaptation on left neglect. Neurology 66:1859–1867
101. Danckert J, Ferber S, Goodale MA (2008) Direct effects of prismatic lenses on visuomotor control: an event-related functional MRI study. Eur J Neurosci 28:1696–1704
102. Luauté J, Schwartz S, Rossetti Y, Spiridon M, Rode G, Boisson D, Vuilleumier P (2009) Dynamic changes in brain activity during prism adaptation. J Neurosci 29:169–178
103. Chapman HL, Eramudugolla R, Gavrilescu M, Strudwick MW, Loftus A, Cunnington R, Mattingley JB (2010) Neural mechanismsunderlying spatial realignment during adaptation to optical wedge prisms. Neuropsychologia 48:2595–2601
104. Pisella L, Mattingley JB (2004) The contribution of spatial remapping impairments to unilateral visual neglect. Neurosci Biobehav Rev 28:181–200

105. Redding GM, Wallace B (2006) Prism adaptation and unilateral neglect: review and analysis. Neuropsychologia 44:1–20
106. Rousseaux M, Bernati T, Saj A, Kozlowski O (2006) Ineffectiveness of prism adaptation on spatial neglect signs. Stroke 37:542–543
107. Schindler I, Kerkhoff G, Karnath HO, Keller I, Goldenberg G (2002) Neck muscle vibration induces lasting recovery in spatial neglect. J Neurol Neurosurg Psychiatry 73:412–419
108. Wiart L, Côme AB, Debelleix X, Petit H, Joseph PA, Mazaux JM, Barat M (1997) Unilateral neglect syndrome rehabilitation by trunk rotation and scanning training. Arch Phys Med Rehabil 78:424–429
109. Polanowska K, Seniow J, Paprot E, Lesniak M, Czlonkowska A (2009) Left-hand somatosensory stimulation combined with visual scanning training in rehabilitation for post-stroke hemineglect: a randomised, double-blind study. Neuropsychol Rehabil 19:364–382
110. Robertson IH, Manly T, Beschin N, Daini R, Haeske-Dewick H, Hömberg V, Jehkonen M, Pizzamiglio G, Shiel A, Weber E (1997) Auditory sustained attention is a marker of unilateral spatial neglect. Neuropsychologia 35:1527–1532
111. Husain M, Shapiro K, Martin J, Kennard C (1997) Abnormal temporal dynamics of visual attention in spatial neglect patients. Nature 385:154–156
112. Battelli L, Cavanagh P, Intriligator J, Tramo MJ, Hénaff MA, Michel F, Barton JJ (2001) Unilateral right parietal damage leads to bilateral deficit for high-level motion. Neuron 32:985–995
113. Doricchi F, Incoccia C (1998) Seeing only the right half of the forest but cutting down all the trees? Nature 394:75–78
114. Husain M, Mannan S, Hodgson T, Wojciulik E, Driver J, Kennard C (2001) Impaired spatial working memory across saccades contributes to abnormal search in parietal neglect. Brain 124:942–952
115. Malhotra P, Jäger HR, Parton A, Greenwood R, Playford ED, Brown MM, Driver J, Husain M (2005) Spatial working memory capacity in unilateral neglect. Brain 128:424–435
116. Robertson IH (2001) Do we need the "lateral" in unilateral neglect? Spatially nonselective attention deficits in unilateral neglect and their implications for rehabilitation. Neuroimage 14:585–590
117. Malhotra P, Parton AD, Greenwood R, Husain M (2006) Noradrenergic modulation of space exploration in visual neglect. Ann Neurol 59:186–190
118. Seron X, Rossetti Y, Vallat-Azouvi C, Pradat-Diehl P, Azouvi P (2008) Cognitive rehabilitation. Rev Neurol 164:S154–S163
119. O'Shea J (2009) Cognitive neurology: stimulating research on neglect. Curr Biol 19:R76–R77
120. Fierro B, Brighina F, Bisiach E (2006) Improving neglect by TMS. Behav Neurol 17:169–176
121. Koch O, Oliveri M, Cheeran B, Ruge D, Lo Gerfo E, Salerno S, Torriero S, Marconi B, Mori F, Driver J, Rothwell JC, Caltagirone C (2008) Hyperexcitability of parietal-motor functional connections in the intact left-hemisphere of patients with neglect. Brain 131:3147–3155
122. Berberovic N, Pisella L, Morris AP, Mattingley JB (2004) Prismatic adaptation reduces biased temporal order judgement in spatial neglect. Neuroreport 15:1199–1204
123. Striemer C, Danckert J (2007) Prism adaptation reduces the disengage deficit in right brain damage patients. Neuroreport 18:99–103
124. Nijboer TC, McIntosh RD, Nys GM, Dijkerman HC, Milner AD (2008) Prism adaptation improves voluntary but not automatic orienting in neglect. Neuroreport 19:293–298
125. Kerkhoff G, Rossetti Y (2006) Plasticity in spatiel neglect: recovery and rehabilitaion Restor Neurol Neurosci 24:201–206
126. Mizuno K, Tsuji T, Takebayashi T, Fujiwara T, Hase K, Liu M. Prism adaptation therapy enhances rehabilitation of stroke patients with unilateral spatial neglect: a randomized, controlled trial. Neurorehabil Neural Repair (in press)

Toward a Cure Based on a Better Understanding of Autism Spectrum Disorder

Shigeru Kitazawa and Tamami Nakano

Abstract Autism is a disorder of neural development characterized by impairments in social cognition and communications. By applying multidimensional scaling to the analysis of temporo-spatial gaze behaviors, we quantitatively demonstrated that normal control participants shared highly stereotypical gaze patterns while viewing socially relevant video stimuli, whereas children and adults with autism spectrum disorders (ASD) were variable in their gaze patterns. Many distant cortical areas has been implicated for such deficits of social ability. From these, we hypothesized that ASD derives from anomalous neural connections in their brain with long-range underconnectivity. In support of the hypothesis, we found a weakness of individuals with ASD in naming familiar objects moved behind a narrow slit, which was worsened by the absence of local salient features. Temporal integration of successive visual information during slit viewing involves a distributed cortical network, including higher visual areas and parietal association areas. Thus, the long-range underconnectivity implicated in the autistic brain may result in a deficit in visual temporal integration across these areas. Understanding how the interconnections are impaired in individuals with ASD is essential for improving present methods for treatment, such as early intensive intervention using applied behavior analysis.

S. Kitazawa (✉)
Department of Neurophysiology, Juntendo University Graduate School of Medicine,
2-1-1 Hongo, Bunkyo-ku, Tokyo 113-8421, Japan
e-mail: kitazawa@juntendo.ac.jp

T. Nakano
Department of Neurophysiology, Juntendo University Graduate School of Medicine,
2-1-1 Hongo, Bunkyo-ku, Tokyo 113-8421, Japan
and
CREST, Japan Science and Technology Agency,
Kawaguchi-shi, Saitama 332-0012, Japan

K. Kansaku and L.G. Cohen (eds.), *Systems Neuroscience and Rehabilitation*,
DOI 10.1007/978-4-431-54008-3_7, © Springer 2011

Introduction

Autistic disorder is, by definition, a developmental disorder characterized by impairments in social interaction, impairments in communication and repetitive behaviors with an onset before the age of three [1]. The prevalence of autism and related spectrum disorders (ASDs) is substantially higher than previously recognized. The prevalence of childhood autism was reported to be about 4 per 1,000 and that of all ASDs was as large as 12 per 1,000 [2]. It is thus an urgent issue for services in health care, social care and education to recognize and meet the needs of children with some form of ASD, who constitutes 1% of the whole population [2].

However, whether the increase is due to better ascertainment, broadening diagnostic criteria, or increased incidence is still unclear. This is because the diagnosis inevitably depends on subjective judgments as to whether each item of diagnostic criteria is met or not. It is therefore important to develop objective measures for evaluating each deficit in different domains. Such objective measures should be useful for evaluating the effects of treatment and intervention as well.

To quantify the deficits in the social domain, we examined temporo-spatial gaze patterns in children and adults with and without ASD while they viewed short video clips [3]. We first present how we were able to quantify unsociability by applying multidimensional scaling to the temporo-spatial gaze patterns.

We then address a deficit in the cognitive domain other than the triad of the diagnostic criteria. Individuals with ASD are hypothesized to show weakness in integrating local elements into a coherent whole [4, 5]. To quantify the deficit in the cognitive domain, we used a naming task of familiar objects moved behind a narrow slit [6].

Quantification of Temporospatial Gaze Patterns

Eye-tracking has been used to investigate gaze behavior in individuals with autism spectral disorder (ASD) while viewing socially salient stimuli like faces [7–11]. Fixation time analysis has been applied in most studies so far, but results have not been consistent (for review see [12]). For example, mouth-viewing in adolescents and young adults with ASD reported in one study [7] was not found when younger children served as subjects [8, 9, 11]. von Hofsten et al. [11] reported that not only preschool children with ASD but also typically developing young children looked at the mouth in most of the time. It is probable that the ratio of eye/mouth viewing behaviors changes with maturation. Studies to date have yet to find characteristic gaze behaviors shared by both children and adults with ASD.

To sort out core gaze behaviors in ASD from those that change with maturation, it is necessary to test both age groups using the same stimuli that could attract both age groups. For this purpose, we examined temporo-spatial gaze patterns in 25 young children with ASD (the mean chronological age, 4:11 years; the mean developmental age, 3:1 years), 25 typically developing children (TD children, mean chronological age 3:1 years), 27 adults with ASD (mean 29.5 y.o.) and 27 normal adults (mean 32 y.o.), while they viewed the same ecological short-lasting video clips taken from films and TV programs for young children.

The video stimulus was 77 s long and consisted of 12 short video clips with sound, each of which lasted for around 6 s. These clips featured one, two, three or more main characters who talked to each other, or to the audience in front of the TV, with varying degrees of social context and distracters in each scene. Gaze positions of both eyes were measured at 50 Hz with a remote eye-tracker (Tobii, x50, Tobii Technology AB).

Multidimensional Scaling

To take all temporo-spatial patterns of gaze from all subjects into account, we summarized the data by using multi-dimensional scaling. In short, we calculated the distance between gaze positions of every pair of subjects ($_{106}C_2$ pairs) at each of 3,850 time points (50 Hz×77 s). Thus 3,850 distances were calculated for each pair of subjects (the i-th and the j-th subjects, for example) and the median of the 3,850 distances was taken as the distance between the i-th and the j-th subjects (d_{ij}). When the pair of subjects looked at the same positions over the 77-s duration, the distance would be zero, for example. By using the distances thus calculated, we defined a between-subject distance matrix to which we applied multidimensional scaling (MDS) to plot each subject on a two-dimensional plane (MDS plane) so that the distance between each pair is reserved as much as possible. If the temporo-spatial gaze trajectories are similar in a pair of subjects, they would be plotted very near to each other, and vice versa. Thus, a group of subjects with a similar gaze behavior would form a cluster on the plane and those with atypical gaze behaviors would be plotted in the periphery, far from the others.

On the MDS plane, normal children (open squares) and normal adults (open circles) distributed near the center forming two distinct clusters (Fig. 1a). In marked contrast, children with ASD (filled squares) and adults with ASD (filled triangles) distributed in the periphery. The MDS distance from the median of the whole distribution (cross) was smaller in the control groups than the ASD groups. A one-way ANOVA revealed a significant main effect of group (F=21.1, p<0.00001), and post-hoc analysis showed significant group differences between the children with ASD and the other groups, and between the adults with ASD and the other groups (Fig. 1b). The results show that normal control groups share similar temporo-spatial gaze patterns, whereas those with ASD show atypical gaze behaviors that are different from one subject to another. A further analysis for the adults with ASD showed that the MDS distance correlated with the autism quotient (AQ) but not with the intelligence quotient (WISC-III), showing that the MDS distance is a good indicator of core symptoms in ASD.

It is also worth noting that both adult groups were distributed in the upper half whereas both children groups in the lower half. A broken line near the x-axis, calculated by applying a linear discriminant analysis, discriminated the children from the adults with an accuracy of more than 95%. All adults (54/54=100%) were plotted

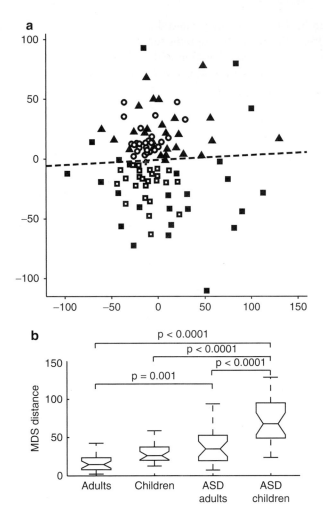

Fig. 1 Temporo-spatial gaze patterns quantified by the full trajectory analysis using multi-dimensional scaling (MDS). (**a**) Distribution of gaze patterns in the MDS plane. Each *symbol* represents a full gaze trajectory (3,728 gaze positions) from a single participant who belonged to the typical adult group (*open circles*), typical child group (*open squares*), adults with ASD group (*filled triangles*) or children with ASD group (*red squares*). A *white cross* indicates the median position of the entire distribution. The *broken line* discriminates adults from children and was calculated using a linear discriminant analysis. (**b**) Group comparison of the MDS distance measured from the cross in (**a**). On each box, the central mark is the median, the edges of the box are the 25th and 75th percentiles and the whiskers extend to the most extreme data points that were not considered outliers if they fell within 1.5 times the box length. Notches in each box show a 95% confidence interval of the median. Reproduced with permission from [3]

above the line and all children except five children with ASD were plotted below (45/50 = 90%). The results suggest that temporo-spatial gaze patterns in normal children develop into those in the adulthood along the line perpendicular to the line of discriminant analysis (dotted line). Although gaze patterns in individuals with

ASD show a wide variation as revealed by their wide distribution in the periphery of the MDS plane, they also share maturation of gaze patterns typically observed in the normal control.

Eye/Mouth Viewing Rate Analysis

Next, we examined if the clear separation of the four groups on the MDS plane was reflected on the difference in the viewing time of the eyes, mouth and the face as a whole. One-way ANOVA and post-hoc tests revealed the following. First, the eye-viewing rate to the total viewing time was longest in normal adults (mean = 44%) and significantly longer than the other three groups: adults with ASD (33%), normal children (33%) and children with ASD (30%).

Second, the mouth-viewing rate was longest in normal children (23%) and significantly longer than the other three groups: children with ASD (13%), normal adults (14%) and adults with ASD (17%). We expected from a previous study [7] that individuals with ASD looks at the mouth longer than normal control at least in adults. The mean viewing rate was indeed longer in adults with ASD (17%) than normal adults (14%), but the difference was not significant. And, to our surprise, the difference was completely reversed in children (normal 23% > ASD 13%).

Third, face-viewing rate was significantly shorter in children with ASD (51%) than the other three groups: normal adults (71%), normal children (69%), and adults with ASD (62%). But, the difference between adults with ASD and normal control was not significant.

Each of the viewing rates showed a significant difference between the adult groups (eye, eye/face; normal > ASD), or between the children groups (mouth, face; normal > ASD) but none of them showed differences common to both age groups.

Frame-by-Frame Analysis

Gaze Alternation During a Scene of Conversation

To identify further which part of the video clips was responsible for the clear between-group differences in distributions on the MDS plane, we carried out frame-by-frame comparisons.

In a 6-s-long clip, two boys talked in turn: the left boy spoke from 1.0 to 1.9 s then the right boy did from 3.7 to 4.8 s. Control groups, both children and adults, showed very stereotyped switches of gaze from one boy to the other. At first, most control subjects viewed the right boy (0.8 s), but at the next moment gazes shifted to the other boy in the left as he spoke "Let's go and see" at 1.9 s (Fig. 2a). In contrast, the gaze positions of adults and children with ASD were scattered widely over the faces and the hands of the two boys (Fig. 2b). At 4.8 s, when most control subjects intensely looked at the face of the right boy (Fig. 2c), adults and children with ASD

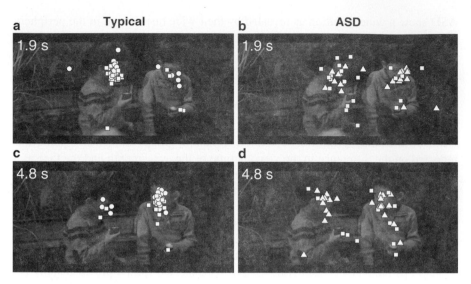

Fig. 2 Frame-by-frame analysis of a clip, in which two boys took turns in a dialogue. (**a**, **b**) Gaze plots of typical adults (*circles*) and children (*squares*) at 1.9 s (**a**) and 4.8 s (**b**) and of adults and children with ASD (*triangles* and *squares*) at 1.9 s (**c**) and 4.8 s (**d**). Reproduced with permission from [3] (color online)

looked widely over the two boys (Fig. 2d). The control subjects shifted their gazes from one subject to another at similar timings but participants with ASD did not share such dynamic temporo-spatial gaze patterns.

Mouth Looking Behavior in TD Children

In another clip (5.5 s in duration), a young girl announced her name. A striking difference between normal children and normal adults appeared, when they looked at the face of the girl who announced her name. The majority of normal children looked at the mouth, whereas the normal adults kept on viewing the eyes (Fig. 3). The results in normal children agree with von Hofsten et al. [11] who showed clear mouth viewing behavior in both 1-year-old (94% of the time) and 3-year-old children (99%) with typical development. We infer that viewing the mouth of a person in speech is a necessary step in normal development that disappears as they grew up into adulthood. This view agrees with a recent finding that greater amounts of fixation to the mother's mouth during live interaction at the age of 6 months predicted higher levels of expressive language at the age of 18 months [13].

Preference to a Telop

In the same clip, a clear group difference appeared when a telop appeared. It is natural that normal children did not shift their gazes to the telop, because most of

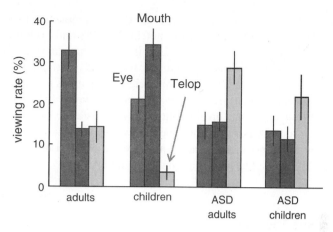

Fig. 3 Group comparisons of the viewing proportions for the eyes (*left*), mouth (*middle*) and the letters in a caption (*right columns*) in a frame of a clip in which a girl announced her name. Reproduced with permission from [3]

them were too young to read (Fig. 3). However, not only adults but also children with ASD, who were impaired even in their speech, showed strong preference to letters in the caption (Fig. 3). This made a marked contrast to normal children and adults who mostly fixated on the face of the girl that was speaking her name. The finding generally agrees with previous literature that reported preference in ASD subjects to non-human objects over human faces [7], preference to non-human sounds over human voices [14].

Autism as an "Anomalous Connection Syndrome"

By applying multidimensional scaling to temporo-spatial gaze patterns, we were successful in finding a quantitative measure (MDS distance) that separated participants with ASD from those with typical development. The MDS distance correlated with the autism quotient (AQ), showing that the MDS distance is a good indicator of core symptoms including social impairments in ASD.

Further post-hoc analyses revealed that children and adults with ASD preferred a telop to a face, and were not good at shifting their gazes from one subject to another at appropriate timings that were shared among control participants.

What are the neural basis for these impairments in social domains? Many areas, such as the orbitofrontal cortex, the anterior cingulate cortex, the fusiform gyrus, the superior temporal sulcus, the amygdala, the inferior frontal gyrus, and the posterior parietal cortex, have been implicated for social impairments [15]. Why are so may areas involved? Recent genetic findings show that many genes encoding neuronal cell-adhesion molecules are involved in ASD [16, 17]. Coupled with emerging anatomical and functional imaging studies [15], it is hypothesized that ASDs many result from structural and functional disconnection of brain regions that are involved in higher-order associations [16, 17]. A neuroanatomical study using MRI

[18] showed that the white matter volume in ASD participants was significantly increased in the radiate compartment but not in the deep and bridging zones: the white matter volume was relatively decreased in the internal capsule, corpus callosum and the basal forebrain. From the findings, we would like to propose that ASDs are characterized by overconnectivity within neighboring areas in addition to underconnectivity between distant areas. Disconnection between distant areas lead to impairments in language that involve anterior and posterior language areas and impairments in social abilities that involve many distant areas. On the other hand, overconnection within neighboring areas may lead to focused interests and repetitive behaviors and special talents sometimes found in ASD.

Deficits in Slit-Viewing

The anomalous connection hypothesis agrees well with the weak central coherence hypothesis proposed by Frith and Happe [4, 5]. Frith and Happe conceptualize a detail-focused cognitive style in ASD as "weak central coherence," implying that an enhancement in local processing derives from a weakness in integrating local elements into a coherent whole. The suggested deficit in central processing in ASD has been challenged [19–21], however, because individuals with ASD are not found to be inferior to normal controls in holistic perception, at least when it is required of them. Results have been inconsistent, even when tasks were designed to make attention to a local feature compete with attention to a global feature, as in Navon hierarchical figures (e.g., an H composed of small Ss) [19]. These reports raise a critical question as to whether the theory of "weak central coherence" is valid at all.

In these previous studies, however, subjects were not required to combine local features to construct a global image of a whole. Rather, they were encouraged to "ignore" local features and attend to the whole. Therefore, no one has directly tested whether individuals with ASD are able to construct a whole image from local features.

To directly examine the ability to integrate elements into a whole image, we asked adults with ASD (n = 17, mean age 32 y.o.) and normal adults (n = 16, mean 29 y.o.) to name a familiar object moving behind a narrow vertical slit [6]. This task benefits from anorthoscopic perception of a visual picture constructed from fragmented pieces of local information [22]. Each subject named 40 figures three times, once for each of three blocks: in the first and the second block, pictures were presented behind the slit (slit-viewing) at a fast and a slow speed, respectively, and in the third block, whole pictures were presented in front of the slit at the fast speed (full-viewing).

In the slit-viewing conditions, the mean rates of correct answers in the ASD group (fast 46%, slow 48%) were strikingly lower than those in the control group (fast 77%, slow 75%) at both speeds. In addition, the rate of correct answers in ASD subjects was lower than that in the control group for every one of the 40 figures. By contrast, both groups successfully named almost all pictures in the full-viewing condition (ASD: 96%, control: 99%). Thus, the ability to identify objects was intact in ASD individuals.

a Group 1: high rate of correct answers in both normal and ASD groups

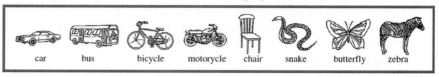

b Group 2: high rate of correct answers in normal group but low rate in ASD group

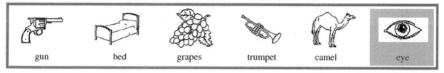

c

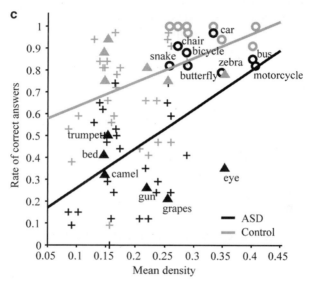

Fig. 4 Object-by-object performance in ASD and control subjects. (**a**) Eight objects that were easily identified by both groups (>75%, Group 1 figures) (**b**) six objects that were easily identified by the control group (>75%), but difficult for the ASD group (Group 2 figures). (**c**) Group comparison of the rate of correct answers (ordinate) relative to the object mean density (abscissa). *Black* and *gray* represent the ASD and control groups, respectively. An analysis of covariance with group as a factor and mean density as a covariate showed significant effects of group ($F_{1,76}=10.4$, $p=0.002$) and their interaction ($F_{2,76}=12.5$, $p<0.0001$). Note a larger slope of the regression line for the ASD group (*black line*; slope=1.8, t=4.3, $p<0.0001$) than for the control group (*gray line*; slope=1.1, t=2.6, $p=0.01$). Reproduced with permission from [6] (color online)

To highlight the relative strengths and weaknesses in the perception of ASD subjects, we further analyzed eight figures that were easy (>75% correct) for both groups to identify (Fig. 4a) and six figures that were easy for the controls but not for the ASD subjects to identify (Fig. 4b; worse than control group rate by >40%). By inspecting these data, we hypothesized that ASD subjects benefited from local salient features (e.g., wheels, stripes of a zebra, textures on the skin surface of a snake), which we quantified by the mean density of the pictures.

This hypothesis is supported by the finding that the rate of correct responses in ASD subjects was more highly dependent on the mean picture density (black symbols in Fig. 4c) as compared to the control group (gray): both groups yielded 80% correct responses at a mean density above 0.3 (circles), but a drop was more apparent in ASD subjects as the mean density decreased to 0.1. Enhancement of the weakness of ASD subjects for a picture that lacked locally salient features indicates that the ASD subjects rely on the local features, although they were clearly instructed to identify the whole picture. Thus, the present results support the original theory of "weak central coherence," which holds that the local bias in ASD subjects reflects a weakness in constructing a coherent whole.

We were successful in detecting this weakness because we did not provide the whole image of the picture at once, but presented each piece of information one-by-one over time. According to recent functional imaging studies, such integration during slit-viewing involves multiple brain areas, including the ventral occipital complex and the human motion complex [23]. In addition, the parietal association cortex might be involved in representing an object image in slit viewing given that brain-damaged patients with unilateral neglect showed contralesional neglect of constructed visual images in slit viewing [24]. Therefore, temporal integration of successive visual information during slit viewing involves a distributed cortical network, including higher visual areas and parietal association areas. Thus, the long-range underconnectivity implicated in the autistic brain [17, 18] may result in a deficit in visual temporal integration across these areas. The results support our hypothesis that ASD is an anomalous connection syndrome.

Toward a Cure Based on a Better Understanding

We hypothesized that ASD is characterized by long-range underconnectivity and short-range overconnectivity in general. However, we should also note that there is a wide range of variability in people with ASD. First of all, ASD include sub-categories like autistic disorder, Asperger syndrome, and pervasive developmental disorder not otherwise specified, depending on the number and combination of core symptoms. Second, some show delayed development from the early period but others develop normally until they are 1 or 2 years old but show regression thereafter. Third, one group of children with ASD responded much better to early behavioral intervention using the techniques of applied behavior analysis than another [25, 26].

It is clear that genetical variability underlies these differences. There are at least 76 genes implicated for ASD [27], and the number is growing day by day. However, no single mutation in a single gene can explain ASD. On the contrary, each represents no more than 1–2% of cases individually [27]. Considering the concordance rate of diagnosis between monozygotic twins (70–90%) and between dizygotic twins (0–10%), mutations of several genes, say around four, are required to manifest ASD. The number of combinations of genes that would lead to ASD is just enormous (e.g., $_{76}C_4 >$ one million). Patterns of deficits in neural connections and the time course of neural development should differ from one child to another. We should somehow figure out causal relationships between quantitative measures in behaviors and neural connectivity among cortical areas, and further relationships with genetics. Classification of ASDs based on these measures is essential for clarifying the causes of ASDs and further to develop effective methods of interventions and therapies for each child and adult with ASD.

References

1. American Psychiatric Association (2000) Diagnostic and statistical manual of mental disorders: DSM-IV-TR, vol 37. American Psychiatric Association, Washington, DC, 943 pp
2. Baird G, Simonoff E, Pickles A, Chandler S, Loucas T, Meldrum D, Charman T (2006) Prevalence of disorders of the autism spectrum in a population cohort of children in South Thames: the special needs and autism project (SNAP). Lancet 368:210–215
3. Nakano T, Tanaka K, Endo Y, Yamane Y, Yamamoto T, Nakano Y, Ohta H, Kato N, Kitazawa S (2010) Atypical gaze patterns in children and adults with autism spectrum disorders dissociated from developmental changes in gaze behaviour. Proc Biol Sci 277:2935–2943
4. Frith U (1989) Autism: explaining the enigma. Blackwell, Oxford, UK
5. Happe F, Frith U (2006) The weak coherence account: detail-focused cognitive style in autism spectrum disorders. J Autism Dev Disord 36:5–25
6. Nakano T, Ota H, Kato N, Kitazawa S (2010) Deficit in visual temporal integration in autism spectrum disorders. Proc Biol Sci 277:1027–1030
7. Klin A, Jones W, Schultz R, Volkmar F, Cohen D (2002) Visual fixation patterns during viewing of naturalistic social situations as predictors of social competence in individuals with autism. Arch Gen Psychiatry 59:809–816
8. van der Geest JN, Kemner C, Camfferman G, Verbaten MN, van Engeland H (2002) Looking at images with human figures: comparison between autistic and normal children. J Autism Dev Disord 32:69–75
9. van der Geest JN, Kemner C, Verbaten MN, van Engeland H (2002) Gaze behavior of children with pervasive developmental disorder toward human faces: a fixation time study. J Child Psychol Psychiatry 43:669–678
10. Dalton KM, Nacewicz BM, Johnstone T, Schaefer HS, Gernsbacher MA, Goldsmith HH, Alexander AL, Davidson RJ (2005) Gaze fixation and the neural circuitry of face processing in autism. Nat Neurosci 8:519–526
11. von Hofsten C, Uhlig H, Adell M, Kochukhova O (2009) How children with autism look at events. Res Autism Spectr Disord 3:556–569
12. Boraston Z, Blakemore SJ (2007) The application of eye-tracking technology in the study of autism. J Physiol 581:893–898
13. Young GS, Merin N, Rogers SJ, Ozonoff S (2009) Gaze behavior and affect at 6 months: predicting clinical outcomes and language development in typically developing infants and infants at risk for autism. Dev Sci 12:798–814
14. Gervais H, Belin P, Boddaert N, Leboyer M, Coez A, Sfaello I, Barthelemy C, Brunelle F, Samson Y, Zilbovicius M (2004) Abnormal cortical voice processing in autism. Nat Neurosci 7:801–802
15. Amaral DG, Schumann CM, Nordahl CW (2008) Neuroanatomy of autism. Trends Neurosci 31:137–145
16. Geschwind DH, Levitt P (2007) Autism spectrum disorders: developmental disconnection syndromes. Curr Opin Neurobiol 17:103–111
17. Wang K, Zhang H, Ma D, Bucan M, Glessner JT, Abrahams BS, Salyakina D, Imielinski M, Bradfield JP, Sleiman PM, Kim CE, Hou C, Frackelton E, Chiavacci R, Takahashi N, Sakurai T,

Rappaport E, Lajonchere CM, Munson J, Estes A, Korvatska O, Piven J, Sonnenblick LI, Alvarez Retuerto AI, Herman EI, Dong H, Hutman T, Sigman M, Ozonoff S, Klin A, Owley T, Sweeney JA, Brune CW, Cantor RM, Bernier R, Gilbert JR, Cuccaro ML, McMahon WM, Miller J, State MW, Wassink TH, Coon H, Levy SE, Schultz RT, Nurnberger JI, Haines JL, Sutcliffe JS, Cook EH, Minshew NJ, Buxbaum JD, Dawson G, Grant SF, Geschwind DH, Pericak-Vance MA, Schellenberg GD, Hakonarson H (2009) Common genetic variants on 5p14.1 associate with autism spectrum disorders. Nature 459:528–533
18. Herbert MR, Ziegler DA, Makris N, Filipek PA, Kemper TL, Normandin JJ, Sanders HA, Kennedy DN, Caviness VS Jr (2004) Localization of white matter volume increase in autism and developmental language disorder. Ann Neurol 55:530–540
19. Plaisted K, Swettenham J, Rees L (1999) Children with autism show local precedence in a divided attention task and global precedence in a selective attention task. J Child Psychol Psychiatry 40:733–742
20. Caron MJ, Mottron L, Berthiaume C, Dawson M (2006) Cognitive mechanisms, specificity and neural underpinnings of visuospatial peaks in autism. Brain 129:1789–1802
21. Mottron L, Dawson M, Soulieres I, Hubert B, Burack J (2006) Enhanced perceptual functioning in autism: an update, and eight principles of autistic perception. J Autism Dev Disord 36:27–43
22. Parks TE (1965) Post-retinal visual storage. Am J Psychol 78:145–147
23. Yin C, Shimojo S, Moore C, Engel SA (2002) Dynamic shape integration in extrastriate cortex. Curr Biol 12:1379–1385
24. Bisiach E, Luzzatti C, Perani D (1979) Unilateral neglect, representational schema and consciousness. Brain 102:609–618
25. Lovaas OI (1987) Behavioral treatment and normal educational and intellectual functioning in young autistic children. J Consult Clin Psychol 55:3–9
26. Sallows GO, Graupner TD (2005) Intensive behavioral treatment for children with autism: four-year outcome and predictors. Am J Ment Retard 110:417–438
27. Abrahams BS, Geschwind DH (2008) Advances in autism genetics: on the threshold of a new neurobiology. Nat Rev Genet 9:341–355

Exceeding the Limits: Behavioral Enhancement Via External Influence

Katsumi Watanabe

Abstract Recent studies in cognitive neuroscience point to the possibility that external factors we are not necessarily aware of can augment our perception, cognition, and actions. This chapter described two examples of behavioral limits being overcome by the use of external factors: (1) transcranial direct current stimulation (tDCS) and (2) behavioral speed contagion. The use of tDCS to improve cognitive and motor function has been increasingly investigated in double-blind sham-controlled studies. The facilitation effects of anodal tDCS may have great potential for enhancement of cognitive and motor function beyond normal limits or in clinical applications for neurorehabilitation. Behavioral speed contagion is an example of unconscious mimicry of an observed behavior, which forces a redefinition of "limits". In a recent study, subjects tended to modify their reaction times according to others' movements, even when the observed and to-be-executed movements were unrelated. The influence of others over our own behaviors can potentially be utilized to exceed our behavioral limits. The two approaches presented in this chapter suggest that external influences should not be avoided but instead studied and used, and that our expected limits can be exceeded.

Introduction

There are several ways to augment our abilities. Learning or training is one method. Using tools is another way to achieve goals beyond our normal capabilities. These approaches have been well examined in both neuroscience and cognitive science.

K. Watanabe (✉)
Research Center for Advanced Science and Technology, The University of Tokyo,
4-6-1, Komaba, Meguro-ku, Tokyo 153-8904, Japan
and
National Institute of Advanced Industrial Science and Technology,
1-1-1, Higashi, Tsukuba, Ibaraki, Japan
e-mail: kw@fennel.rcast.u-tokyo.ac.jp

K. Kansaku and L.G. Cohen (eds.), *Systems Neuroscience and Rehabilitation*,
DOI 10.1007/978-4-431-54008-3_8, © Springer 2011

In addition to these ordinary means, the possibility of augmenting sensory, perceptual, cognitive, and motor abilities by using external inputs has also been investigated. This chapter will discuss two instances in which our behavioral limits are overcome by the use of external factors.

The first approach is transcranial direct current stimulation (tDCS), a procedure for cortical stimulation that employs weak direct currents to polarize target brain regions. Depending on the polarity of stimulation, anodal and cathodal tDCS can increase or decrease cortical excitability, respectively, in stimulated brain regions. tDCS has been used increasingly in recent years to investigate human cognitive and motor function in both healthy volunteers and neurological patients. The effects of anodal tDCS on facilitating motor and cognitive functions may have great potential for cognitive and motor enhancement, for example to support learning in healthy volunteers and to speed up rehabilitation in neurological patients.

The second approach, behavioral contagion, is based on the unconscious tendency of people to mimic the behaviors of others, a trend which has been widely documented. Choosing an appropriate category of action and executing it with the appropriate timing are both crucial to the coordination of our actions with those of others. Recently, we conducted a study demonstrating that people tend to modify the timing of their movements according to others' movements even when the observed and to-be-executed movements are unrelated. This finding suggests that behavioral tempo may be contagious: the speed of others' movements may automatically influence the timing of an observer's execution of movement. Even for the simplest movement, we unconsciously adjust our movement speed to those of others, and these unconscious alterations may accumulate to define the limit of behavioral speed.

Transcranial Direct Current Stimulation to Enhance Cognitive Function

Our mental activity and behaviors are governed by neural activity, which is essentially comprised of electrical signals. Therefore, electrical modulations from outside of the brain can alter neutral activity and, potentially, mental processes. Since the skull and other surrounding tissues have high electrical resistance, a strong current has been assumed to be necessary for the induction of any effects on neural activities and consequential mental and behavioral processes. However, accumulating evidence has indicated that tDCS can evoke transient changes in neural activity even with direct current less than 1 mA [1–7].

Clinical applications of direct current electrical stimulation of humans can be dated back to the nineteenth century. In 1960s, studies using both animals and humans were performed [3, 8], but their conclusions were mixed, which led to progressively fewer studies conducted in the 1970s. However, since the effects of transcranial magnetic stimulation (TMS) were found to confirm the effects of direct stimulation of motor cortex in the mid-1980s, interest in tDCS has again increased. First, Priori et al. (1998) reported an increase in the excitability of stimulated cortical regions [1], and subsequent systematic investigation by Nitsche et al. (2000) brought renewed attention to the effects of tDCS on the nervous system [2].

tDCS is a simple technique that stimulates brain regions by delivering weak direct currents through the skull. One interesting property of tDCS is that, depending on the polarity of stimulation, it can increase (anodal tDCS) or decrease (cathodal tDCS) the excitability of a stimulated cortical region, which allows us to investigate causal relationships between brain activity and behavior. The excitability of the hand motor cortex, for example, is transiently increased by anodal tDCS and decreased by cathodal tDCS [2, 9, 10]. Anodal tDCS of motor cortex enhanced the motor-evoked potentials (MEP) induced by TMS, and cathodal tDCS suppressed MEPs [2, 9]. Although the mechanisms by which tDCS affects neural activity in human motor cortex are still unknown, tDCS appears to alter the membrane potential of groups of neurons, as opposed to TMS, which induces neuronal spikes. Animal studies have demonstrated that anodal tDCS depolarizes resting membrane potential (and consequently increases spontaneous spike discharges), whereas cathodal tDCS hyperpolarizes it (and decreases spontaneous spike discharges) [11–13].

Compared with other brain stimulation techniques, a tDCS device is relatively small and elicits no acoustic noise or muscle twitching, making it suitable for double-blind sham-controlled studies and clinical applications [6, 14, 15]. Furthermore, tDCS-induced changes in excitability are associated with changes in the performance of both cognitive and motor tasks [3, 4, 16]. The facilitation effects of anodal tDCS on motor and cognitive functions have motivated researchers to examine the effects of tDCS in a wide range of applications. The following sections will summarize recent reports on tDCS effects on cognitive and behavioral functions (see [3] for a review of studies prior to [1]).

Anodal tDCS has been shown to enhance motor functions. The application of anodal tDCS to the hand motor cortex was associated with a temporary improvement in the performance of hand motor tasks mimicking activities of daily living (Jebsen-Taylor hand function test) [17]. We recently examined whether anodal tDCS over the leg motor cortex could facilitate the performance of leg motor tasks involving pinch force and reaction time [18]. Subjects performed the tasks before, during, and after anodal, cathodal, or sham tDCS over the leg motor cortex. Anodal tDCS transiently enhanced maximal leg pinch force but not reaction time during its application. Cathodal and sham stimulation had no effect on performance. No interventions affected hand pinch force or reaction time, indicating that the effect of tDCS was spatially specific (Fig. 1). Other studies have also reported that tDCS influences motor learning [19, 20]. Nietzsche et al. (2003) demonstrated that anodal tDCS of motor cortex enhances sequential motor learning, whereas no effect was observed with tDCS of premotor cortex or frontal cortex [21]. In another study, anodal tDCS improved the early stage of learning in a visuo-motor tracking task [22].

Sensory and perceptual functions can also be influenced by tDCS in a polarity-dependent manner. The application of cathodal tDCS to the somatosensory cortex

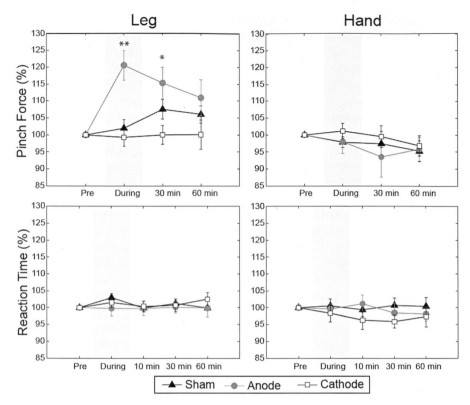

Fig. 1 The effect of tDCS on pinch force and reaction time. Mean performance is plotted as a function of time relative to the intervention. Data is normalized with respect to pre-intervention baseline values. During and 30 min after application of anodal tDCS (*grey circles*), maximal pinch force increased compared to baseline. Cathodal (*white rectangle*) and sham (*black triangle*) stimulation had no effect on maximal pinch force. Anodal and cathodal tDCS had no effect on leg reaction time, hand pinch force, or hand reaction time. Reproduced with modification from Tanaka et al. [18] with permission

has been reported to temporarily decrease performance in a tactile discrimination task [23]. In contrast, application of anodal tDCS increased tactile performance [24]. Studies have also reported that tDCS of somatosensory cortex influences the amplitude and frequency power of somatosensory evoked potentials [25, 26]. With regard to visual function, Antal et al. (2001) reported that cathodal tDCS of primary visual cortex temporarily decreased the luminance contrast threshold compared with anodal tDCS [27]. Anodal tDCS of primary visual cortex also enhanced TMS-induced phosphene, which was weakened by cathodal tDCS [28, 29]. Likewise, the N70 component of visual evoked potentials could be enhanced by anodal tDCS and suppressed by cathodal tDCS [30]. tDCS has also been reported to influence higher visual functions [31, 32].

Anodal tDCS of the left frontal cortex was reported to enhance the performance of tasks that require working memory [33–35]. On the other hand, tDCS has also complex, mainly suppressive effects on working memory when it is applied to the cerebellum [36] or to the frontal cortex of both hemispheres [37]. This suppressive effect does not appear to be polarity specific, which remains to be clarified. Sleep, in particular non-rapid eye movement (REM) sleep, has been implicated in the process of memory consolidation [38–40]. Marshall et al. (2004, 2006) applied anodal tDCS to the frontal cortex of human subjects in the period of non-REM sleep and found that memory performance for paired word association was significantly enhanced [41, 42].

In a recent study, anodal tDCS of Wernicke's area enhanced performance in a picture-naming task [43]. Fecteau et al. (2007) have examined the effect of tDCS on decision making under uncertainty [44]. In the experiment, the subjects inflated a balloon presented on a computer monitor by pressing a button. Each button press resulted in a 5-cent reward, but the balloon was broken if its capacity, which was unknown to the subject, was exceeded. When the frontal cortices of both hemispheres were stimulated with tDCS, the subjects tended to avoid high-risk choices and choose not to press the button. Since this effect did not depend on the polarity-hemisphere combination, the authors speculated that inter-hemispheric balance is important for decision making under uncertainty. A similar finding has been reported in a gambling task [45]. Anodal tDCS also has been reported to enhance a probabilistic classification task [46].

Since tDCS began as a clinical practice, it is natural and important to examine possible applications of tDCS to neuro-rehabilitation. Several studies have investigated the therapeutic effects of tDCS on motor dysfunction after stroke. Anodal tDCS of the hand motor cortex increased stroke patients' maximal pinch force, shortened their reaction time for performing simple hand motor tasks [47, 48], and enhanced performance on the Jebsen-Taylor hand function test [17, 49, 50]. Our recent study of tDCS effects on leg motor function also supports the usefulness of tDCS in neuro-rehabilitation [51]. In addition to stroke patients, the effect of tDCS has also been tested on motor dysfunctions in Parkinson's disease [52] and in focal dystonia.

Neuro-rehabilitation of aphasic patients is another possible application of tDCS. Monti et al. (2008) reported that cathodal tDCS of Wernicke's area increased the performance of aphasic patients in a picture-naming task [53]. Additionally, tDCS has been suggested to alter preference and/or craving behaviors. For example, bilateral tDCS of frontal cortex has been reported to alter preference in patients with addictive disorders and to reduce alcohol craving [54], smoking craving [55], and craving for specific foods [56]. Thus, tDCS appears to be highly applicable to a wide range of neuronal dysfunctions and a useful tool for neuro-rehabilitation.

Behavioral Contagion

People imitate each other. Casual observations suggest that long-term relationships make a husband and wife look and behave similarly. Emulation of others is not limited to conscious behaviors. People also unintentionally mimic others' behaviors (the "chameleon effect") [57]. The existence of unconscious behavioral imitations supports the hypothesis that essential links exist between perception and action [58–60]; the processes of perceiving, preparing, and executing actions may inevitably interact or even overlap.

The identification of "mirror neurons" in the monkey ventral cortex has further increased out understanding of action–perception coupling. Mirror neurons fire not only when the observer produces certain actions but also when the observer see others performing the same goal-directed actions (e.g., [61, 62]). The existence of a similar system has been suggested by human brain imaging studies of mirror neuron systems (e.g., [63]). Although various functions have been speculated for the mirror neuron system including understanding the actions of others, observational learning by imitation, empathy, and language [64], no clear consensus has been reached.

However, the mirror neuron system clearly predicts that the execution and observation of an action may mutually interact. Several studies have demonstrated that the execution (and preparation) of actions alters subjects' perception of the action when performed by others (e.g., [65, 66]). For example, Casile and Geise (2006) found that non-visual motor training influences visual motion perception [65]. Similarly, observing the actions of others affects the observer's execution of actions. While observing an action, motor-evoked potentials from the hand muscles that a subject would use in executing the action significantly increase [67] in a manner that is temporally linked to the observed movement [68]. Movement observation has also been shown to affect movement execution in a simple response task [69]. Additionally, seeing actions performed by others expedites or impedes the execution of an action, as measured by reaction time, depending on whether it is similar or dissimilar to the observed action [69–72]. For example, visual presentation of a different hand position significantly slowed reaction time to initiate a finger movement or grasp an object compared to presentation of a similar hand position [70]. These findings hold true even when the movement observation is task irrelevant.

Behavioral contagion (or the "chameleon effect" [57]) of actions, such as that evidenced by the mirror neuron system and the above behavioral studies, may have some function in promoting communication and understanding the mental states of others [73, 74] as well as in coordinating actions with others [75, 76]. Efficient communication and joint action require sharing and/or adjusting behavioral tempo according to others.

In a recent study [77], we examined the possibility of behavioral speed contagion by utilizing point-light biological motion stimuli [78]. People can readily recognize actions in biological motion displays even though visual information (particularly form cues) is greatly reduced [79–81]. In the experiment, participants observed point-light biological motion sequences that represented various actions (Fig. 2a; e.g., [82, 83]). The biological motion displays were played at three different speeds: the original speed (the same speed as recorded), double speed, or half speed. After a delay period from the termination of the biological motion stimulus, the fixation cross underwent a small change to which the observers responded as quickly as possible by button press. Our results indicated that observing faster or slower biological motions produced faster or slower responses, respectively (Fig. 3). Notably, the biological motions were observed before the task, and they were irrelevant

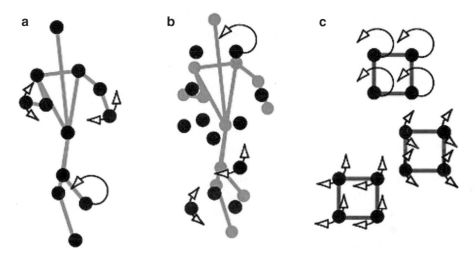

Fig. 2 (**a**) Biological motion stimuli. (**b**) Scrambled motion stimuli were created by randomizing the dot starting positions that defined the biological motion randomly chosen for each trial. (**c**) To generate object motion stimuli, four *black dots* were placed at the corners of three imaginary squares positioned at random locations within an imaginary rectangle, and the three imaginary squares were moved along randomly selected biological motion trajectories. The use of biological motion stimuli is advantageous in that it allows scrambled motion, in which control stimuli are generated by randomizing the starting positions of the dots. Scrambled motion (**b**) renders a stimulus meaningless while ensuring that the local motion cues are identical to the original biological motion (**a**). Reproduced from Watanabe [77] with permission

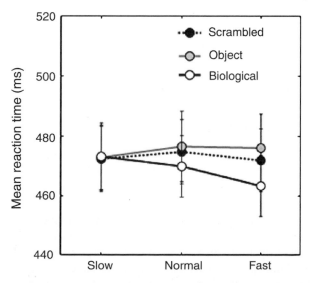

Fig. 3 Reaction time demonstrated a trend to decrease with presentation speed in the biological motion condition, but no such trend was observed in the scrambled and object motion conditions. Reproduced with modification from Watanabe [77] with permission

to the task. In addition, the speed contagion appeared to occur only within 1 s after biological motion had ended [77], which indicates that the underlying mechanism is based on automatic, rather than deliberative, processes. Furthermore, this automatic behavioral speed contagion was not observed with "scrambled" or "object" motion sequences (Fig. 3), highlighting the importance of "social" rather than "physical" environment.

Speed contagion may differ from conventional movement facilitations by observation because it is not specific to the action category performed by others. Observing an action has been reported to facilitate similar actions and impede dissimilar actions [69–72], and neurophysiological studies have corroborated behavioral findings (motor-evoked potential, [68, 84]; brain imaging studies, [62, 63, 85]. In behavioral speed contagion, the stimulus observed and the movement to be performed do not need to be similar; nevertheless, reaction times tend to be shorter or longer after observing the fast or slow actions, respectively. In this regard, speed contagion may be more closely related to higher-level social priming or the "chameleon effect" [57]. For example, a tendency for people to behave more slowly after exposed to stereotyped words semantically related to the elderly has been demonstrated [86].

Although the precise mechanism underlying speed contagion is not known, the modulation of movement timing by observation may be of possible functional significance. The coordination of our actions with those of others is critical to efficient communication [75]. Shared action representation and the modeling of others' performance in relation to one's own are necessary for the successful coordination of action in a social context, which requires speed tuning and synchronization of our actions with those of others. Conversely, perhaps, our limit to behavioral speed could possibly be overcome simply by exposing ourselves to a particular social environment.

Another implication of speed contagion, or behavioral contagion in general, is that limits that we tend to believe are due to physical or neural constraints may be psychological and/or social constraints. The reaction time in the normal speed condition [77] is considered to be the behavioral limit in everyday life. The action is so simple that we think we cannot press the button faster. Nonetheless, just observing others' actions at a tempo faster than usual helped participants react faster and exceed their own limits. Thus, our behavior is under constant tuning by others, and our abilities can be determined only when the social contexts are defined.

Conclusion

Recent studies in cognitive neuroscience point to the possibility that augmenting our perception, cognition, and action is possible by means of external factors that we are not necessarily aware of. Studies of human cognitive and motor function in both healthy volunteers and neurological patients have increasingly used tDCS for double-blind sham-controlled studies and clinical applications. The facilitation effects on motor and cognitive functions by anodal tDCS may have great potential for cognitive and motor enhancement, for example to support learning in healthy volunteers and to expedite the rehabilitation process in neurological patients.

Although the neural processes underlying speed contagion remain unclear, the phenomenon has led us rethink "limits". Our abilities are constrained by multiple factors, among which the influence of other people cannot be bypassed. In other words, understanding and utilizing the influence of others could be one potential way to exceed our limits. The two approaches presented in this chapter suggest that external influences should not be avoided but rather utilized, with the aim of advancing neurological performance and recovery beyond currently expected limits.

Acknowledgements This chapter is based on a talk at the Conference on Systems Neuroscience and Rehabilitation held in Tokorozawa City in March 2010. Some of the materials used are based on other materials [16, 18, 51, 77]. The writing of this chapter was supported by Japan Science and Technology Agency. The author would like to thank Dr. Satoshi Tanaka for helpful comments. Special thanks are due to Dr. Kenji Kansaku for organizing the fruitful workshop.

References

1. Priori A, Berardelli A, Rona S, Accornero N, Manfredi M (1998) Polarization of the human motor cortex through the scalp. Neuroreport 9:2257–2260
2. Nitsche MA, Paulus W (2000) Excitability changes induced in the human motor cortex by weak transcranial direct current stimulation. J Physiol 527:633–639
3. Priori A (2003) Brain polarization in humans: a reappraisal of an old tool for prolonged non-invasive modulation of brain excitability. Clin Neurophysiol 114:589–595
4. Wassermann EM, Grafman J (2005) Recharging cognition with DC brain polarization. Trends Cogn Sci 9:503–505
5. Antal A, Nitsche MA, Paulus W (2006) Transcranial direct current stimulation and the visual cortex. Brain Res Bull 68:459–463
6. Fregni F, Pascual-Leone A (2007) Technology insight: noninvasive brain stimulation in neurology-perspectives on the therapeutic potential of rTMS and tDCS. Nat Clin Pract Neurol 3:383–393
7. Sparing R, Mottaghy FM (2008) Noninvasive brain stimulation with transcranial magnetic or direct current stimulation (TMS/tDCS) – from insights into human memory to therapy of its dysfunction. Methods 44:329–337
8. Zago S, Ferrucci R, Fregni F, Priori A (2008) Bartholow, Sciamanna, Alberti: pioneers in the electrical stimulation of the exposed human cerebral cortex. Neuroscientist 14:521–528
9. Nitsche MA, Paulus W (2001) Sustained excitability elevations induced by transcranial DC motor cortex stimulation in humans. Neurology 57:1899–1901
10. Furubayashi T, Terao Y, Arai N, Okabe S, Mochizuki H, Hanajima R, Hamada M, Yugeta A, Inomata-Terada S, Ugawa Y (2008) Short and long duration transcranial direct current stimulation (tDCS) over the human hand motor area. Exp Brain Res 185:279–286
11. Bindman LJ, Lippold OC, Redfearn JW (1962) Long-lasting changes in the level of the electrical activity of the cerebral cortex produced by polarizing currents. Nature 196:584–585
12. Bindman LJ, Lippold OC, Redfearn JW (1964) The action of brief polarizing currents on the cerebral cortex of the rat (1) during current flow and (2) in the production of long-lasting after-effects. J Physiol 172:369–382
13. Creutzfeldt OD, Fromm GH, Kapp H (1962) Influence of transcortical d-c currents on cortical neuronal activity. Exp Neurol 5:436–452
14. Gandiga PC, Hummel FC, Cohen LG (2006) Transcranial DC stimulation (tDCS): a tool for double-blind sham-controlled clinical studies in brain stimulation. Clin Neurophysiol 117:845–850
15. Hummel FC, Cohen LG (2006) Non-invasive brain stimulation: a new strategy to improve neurorehabilitation after stroke? Lancet Neurol 5:708–712

16. Tanaka S, Watanabe K (2009) Transcranial direct current stimulation – a new tool for human cognitive neuroscience. Brain Nerve 61:53–64
17. Fregni F, Boggio PS, Mansur CG, Wagner T, Ferreira MJ, Lima MC, Rigonatti SP, Marcolin MA, Freedman SD, Nitsche MA, Pascual-Leone A (2005) Transcranial direct current stimulation of the unaffected hemisphere in stroke patients. Neuroreport 16:1551–1555
18. Tanaka S, Hanakawa T, Honda M, Watanabe K (2009) Enhancement of pinch force in the lower leg by anodal transcranial direct current stimulation. Exp Brain Res 196:459–465
19. Rosenkranz K, Nitsche MA, Tergau F, Paulus W (2000) Diminution of training-induced transient motor cortex plasticity by weak transcranial direct current stimulation in the human. Neurosci Lett 296:61–63
20. Classen J, Liepert J, Wise SP, Hallett M, Cohen LG (1998) Rapid plasticity of human cortical movement representation induced by practice. J Neurophysiol 79:1117–1123
21. Nitsche MA, Schauenburg A, Lang N, Liebetanz D, Exner C, Paulus W, Tergau F (2003) Facilitation of implicit motor learning by weak transcranial direct current stimulation of the primary motor cortex in the human. J Cogn Neurosci 15:619–626
22. Antal A, Nitsche MA, Kincses TZ, Kruse W, Hoffmann KP, Paulus W (2004) Facilitation of visuo-motor learning by transcranial direct current stimulation of the motor and extrastriate visual areas in humans. Eur J Neurosci 19:2888–2892
23. Rogalewski A, Breitenstein C, Nitsche MA, Paulus W, Knecht S (2004) Transcranial direct current stimulation disrupts tactile perception. Eur J Neurosci 20:313–316
24. Ragert P, Vandermeeren Y, Camus M, Cohen LG (2008) Improvement of spatial tactile acuity by transcranial direct current stimulation. Clin Neurophysiol 119:805–811
25. Dieckhöfer A, Waberski TD, Nitsche M, Paulus W, Buchner H, Gobbelé R (2006) Transcranial direct current stimulation applied over the somatosensory cortex – differential effect on low and high frequency SEPs. Clin Neurophysiol 117:2221–2227
26. Matsunaga K, Nitsche MA, Tsuji S, Rothwell JC (2004) Effect of transcranial DC sensorimotor cortex stimulation on somatosensory evoked potentials in humans. Clin Neurophysiol 115:456–460
27. Antal A, Nitsche MA, Paulus W (2001) External modulation of visual perception in humans. Neuroreport 12:3553–3555
28. Antal A, Kincses TZ, Nitsche MA, Paulus W (2003) Manipulation of phosphene thresholds by transcranial direct current stimulation in man. Exp Brain Res 150:375–378
29. Antal A, Kincses TZ, Nitsche MA, Paulus W (2003) Modulation of moving phosphene thresholds by transcranial direct current stimulation of V1 in human. Neuropsychologia 41:1802–1807
30. Antal A, Kincses TZ, Nitsche MA, Bartfai O, Paulus W (2004) Excitability changes induced in the human primary visual cortex by transcranial direct current stimulation: direct electrophysiological evidence. Invest Ophthalmol Vis Sci 45:702–707
31. Antal A, Varga ET, Nitsche MA, Chadaide Z, Paulus W, Kovács G, Vidnyánszky Z (2004) Direct current stimulation over MT+/V5 modulates motion aftereffect in humans. Neuroreport 15:2491–2494
32. Schweid L, Rushmore RJ, Valero-Cabre A (2008) Cathodal transcranial direct current stimulation on posterior parietal cortex disrupts visuo-spatial processing in the contralateral visual field. Exp Brain Res 186:409–417
33. Fregni F, Boggio PS, Nitsche M, Bermpohl F, Antal A, Feredoes E, Marcolin MA, Rigonatti SP, Silva MT, Paulus W, Pascual-Leone A (2005) Anodal transcranial direct current stimulation of prefrontal cortex enhances working memory. Exp Brain Res 166:23–30
34. Ohn SH, Park CI, Yoo WK, Ko MH, Choi KP, Kim GM, Lee YT, Kim YH (2008) Time-dependent effect of transcranial direct current stimulation on the enhancement of working memory. Neuroreport 19:43–47
35. Boggio PS, Ferrucci R, Rigonatti SP, Covre P, Nitsche M, Pascual-Leone A, Fregni F (2006) Effects of transcranial direct current stimulation on working memory in patients with Parkinson's disease. J Neurol Sci 249:31–38

36. Ferrucci R, Marceglia S, Vergari M, Cogiamanian F, Mrakic-Sposta S, Mameli F, Zago S, Barbieri S, Priori A (2008) Cerebellar transcranial direct current stimulation impairs the practice-dependent proficiency increase in working memory. J Cogn Neurosci 20:1687–1697
37. Marshall L, Molle M, Siebner HR, Born J (2005) Bifrontal transcranial direct current stimulation slows reaction time in a working memory task. BMC Neurosci 6:23
38. Maquet P (2001) The role of sleep in learning and memory. Science 294:1048–1052
39. Gais S, Plihal W, Wagner U, Born J (2000) Early sleep triggers memory for early visual discrimination skills. Nat Neurosci 3:1335–1339
40. Plihal W, Born J (1999) Effects of early and late nocturnal sleep on priming and spatial memory. Psychophysiology 36:571–582
41. Marshall L, Molle M, Hallschmid M, Born J (2004) Transcranial direct current stimulation during sleep improves declarative memory. J Neurosci 24:9985–9992
42. Marshall L, Helgadóttir H, Mölle M, Born J (2006) Boosting slow oscillations during sleep potentiates memory. Nature 444:610–613
43. Sparing R, Dafotakis M, Meister IG, Thirugnanasambandam N, Fink GR (2008) Enhancing language performance with non-invasive brain stimulation – a transcranial direct current stimulation study in healthy humans. Neuropsychologia 46:261–268
44. Fecteau S, Pascual-Leone A, Zald DH, Liguori P, Théoret H, Boggio PS, Fregni F (2007) Activation of prefrontal cortex by transcranial direct current stimulation reduces appetite for risk during ambiguous decision making. J Neurosci 27:6212–6218
45. Fecteau S, Knoch D, Fregni F, Sultani N, Boggio P, Pascual-Leone A (2007) Diminishing risk-taking behavior by modulating activity in the prefrontal cortex: a direct current stimulation study. J Neurosci 27:12500–12505
46. Kincses TZ, Antal A, Nitsche MA, Bártfai O, Paulus W (2004) Facilitation of probabilistic classification learning by transcranial direct current stimulation of the prefrontal cortex in the human. Neuropsychologia 42:113–117
47. Hummel F, Cohen LG (2005) Improvement of motor function with noninvasive cortical stimulation in a patient with chronic stroke. Neurorehabil Neural Repair 19:14–19
48. Hummel FC, Voller B, Celnik P, Floel A, Giraux P, Gerloff C, Cohen LG (2006) Effects of brain polarization on reaction times and pinch force in chronic stroke. BMC Neurosci 7:73
49. Hummel F, Celnik P, Giraux P, Floel A, Wu WH, Gerloff C, Cohen LG (2005) Effects of non-invasive cortical stimulation on skilled motor function in chronic stroke. Brain 128: 490–499
50. Boggio PS, Nunes A, Rigonatti SP, Nitsche MA, Pascual-Leone A, Fregni F (2007) Repeated sessions of noninvasive brain DC stimulation is associated with motor function improvement in stroke patients. Restor Neurol Neurosci 25:123–129
51. Tanaka S, Takeda K, Otaka Y, Kita K, Osu R, Honda M, Sadato N, Hanakawa T, Watanabe K (2011) Single session of transcranial direct current stimulation transiently increases knee extensor force in patients with hemiparetic stroke. Neurorehabil Neural Repair. doi:10.1177/1545968311402091, March 24 [E-pub ahead of print]
52. Fregni F, Boggio PS, Santos MC, Lima M, Vieira AL, Rigonatti SP, Silva MT, Barbosa ER, Nitsche MA, Pascual-Leone A (2006) Noninvasive cortical stimulation with transcranial direct current stimulation in Parkinson's disease. Mov Disord 21:1693–1702
53. Monti A, Cogiamanian F, Marceglia S, Ferrucci R, Mameli F, Mrakic-Sposta S, Vergari M, Zago S, Priori A (2008) Improved naming after transcranial direct current stimulation in aphasia. J Neurol Neurosurg Psychiatry 79:451–453
54. Boggio PS, Sultani N, Fecteau S, Merabet L, Mecca T, Pascual-Leone A, Basaglia A, Fregni F (2008) Prefrontal cortex modulation using transcranial DC stimulation reduces alcohol craving: a double-blind, sham-controlled study. Drug Alcohol Depend 92:55–60
55. Fregni F, Liguori P, Fecteau S, Nitsche MA, Pascual-Leone A, Boggio PS (2008) Cortical stimulation of the prefrontal cortex with transcranial direct current stimulation reduces cue-provoked smoking craving: a randomized, sham-controlled study. J Clin Psychiatry 69:32–40

56. Fregni F, Orsati F, Pedrosa W, Fecteau S, Tome FA, Nitsche MA, Mecca T, Macedo EC, Pascual-Leone A, Boggio PS (2008) Transcranial direct current stimulation of the prefrontal cortex modulates the desire for specific foods. Appetite 51:34–41

57. Chartrand TL, Bargh JA (1999) The chameleon effect: the perception-behavior link and social interaction. J Pers Soc Psychol 76:893–910

58. James W (1890) Principle of psychology. Holt, New York

59. Jeannerod M (1994) The representing brain: neural correlates of motor intention and imagery. Behav Brain Sci 17:187–202

60. Prinz W (1997) Perception and action planning. Eur J Cogn Psychol 9:129–154

61. di Pellegrino G, Fadiga L, Fogassi L, Gallese V, Rizzolatti G (1992) Understanding motor events: a neurophysiological study. Exp Brain Res 91:176–180

62. Rizzolatti G, Fadiga L, Gallese V, Fogassi L (1996) Premotor cortex and the recognition of motor actions. Cogn Brain Res 3:131–141

63. Iacoboni M, Woods RP, Brass M, Bekkering H, Mazziotta JC, Rizzolatti G (1999) Cortical mechanisms of human imitation. Science 286:2526–2528

64. Rizzolatti G, Craighero L (2004) The mirror-neuron system. Annu Rev Neurosci 27:167–192

65. Casile A, Giese MA (2006) Nonvisual motor training influences biological motion perception. Curr Biol 16:69–74

66. Wilson M, Knoblich G (2005) The case for motor involvement in perceiving conspecifics. Psychol Bull 131:460–473

67. Fadiga L, Fogassi L, Pavesi G, Rizzolatti G (1995) Motor facilitation during action observation: a magnetic stimulation study. J Neurophysiol 73:2608–2611

68. Gangitano M, Mottaghy FM, Pascal-Leone A (2001) Phase-specific modulation of cortical motor output during movement observation. Neuroreport 12:1489–1492

69. Brass M, Bekkering H, Prinz W (2001) Movement observation affects movement execution in a simple response task. Acta Psychol 106:3–22

70. Craighero L, Bello A, Fadiga L, Rizzolatti G (2002) Hand action preparation influences the responses to hand pictures. Neuropsychologia 40:492–502

71. Stürmer B, Aschersleben G, Prinz W (2000) Correspondence effects with manual gestures and postures: a study of imitation. J Exp Psychol Hum Percept Perform 26:1746–1759

72. Heyes C, Bird G, Johnson H, Haggard P (2005) Experience modulates automatic imitation. Cogn Brain Res 22:233–240

73. Blackmore SJ, Decety J (2001) From the perception of action to the understanding of intention. Nat Rev Neurosci 2:561–567

74. Wolpert DM, Doya K, Kawato M (2003) A unifying computational framework for motor control and social interaction. Philos Trans R Soc Lond B Biol Sci 358:593–602

75. Sebanz N, Bekkering H, Knoblich G (2006) Joint action: bodies and minds moving together. Trends Cogn Sci 10:70–76

76. Knoblich G, Sebanz N (2006) The social nature of perception and action. Curr Dir Psychol Sci 15:99–104

77. Watanabe K (2008) Behavioral speed contagion: automatic modulation of movement timing by observation of body movements. Cognition 106:1514–1524

78. Johansson G (1973) Visual perception of biological motion and a model for its analysis. Percept Psychophys 14:201–211

79. Thornton IM, Pinto J, Shiffrar M (1998) The visual perception of human locomotion. Cogn Neuropsychol 15:535–552

80. Verfaillie K (2000) Perceiving human locomotion: priming effects in direction discrimination. Brain Cogn 44:192–213

81. Giese MA, Poggio T (2003) Neural mechanisms for the recognition of biological movements. Nat Rev Neurosci 4:179–192

82. Grossman E, Donnelly M, Price R, Pickens D, Morgan V, Neighbor G, Blake R (2000) Brain areas involved in perception of biological motion. J Cogn Neurosci 12:711–720

83. Ikeda H, Blake R, Watanabe K (2005) Eccentric perception of biological motion in unscalably poor. Vision Res 45:1935–1943
84. Fadiga L, Craighero L, Olivier E (2005) Human motor cortex excitability during the perception of others' action. Curr Opin Neurobiol 15:213–218
85. Buccino G, Binkofski F, Fink GR, Fadiga L, Fogassi L, Gallese V, Seitz RJ, Zilles K, Rizzolatti G, Freund HJ (2001) Action observation activates premotor and parietal areas in a somatotopic manner: an fMRI study. Eur J Neurosci 13:400–404
86. Bargh JA, Chen M, Burrows L (1996) Automaticity of social behavior: direct effects of trait construct and stereotype activation on action. J Pers Soc Psychol 71:230–234

References

Neural Correlates of Reasoning by Exclusion

Akitoshi Ogawa

When asked to select a label for a novel object from a given group of labels that includes both novel and familiar labels, one tends to choose a novel label. Nonhuman animals robustly fail to demonstrate the same tendency, although this tendency called "exclusion" that can bias human behavior may seem quite natural. The functional magnetic resonance imaging study described here investigated the neural correlates of this bias. The subjects were trained on two sample-to-comparison associations. In the scanner, they were shown a novel sample and were asked to choose between a trained comparison and a novel comparison. The subjects readily chose the novel comparison and rejected the trained one, thus demonstrating exclusion. Significant activation was observed in the prefrontal cortex (PFC) and inferior parietal lobule (IPL) during exclusion. Medial frontal activation was also observed when the novel stimuli appeared. These results suggest that the medial frontal cortex is associated with novelty detection and that the PFC and IPL are involved in rejecting the defined comparison.

Introduction

> When you have eliminated the impossible, whatever remains, however improbable, must be the truth.
>
> Sherlock Holmes

When confronted with a novel situation and forced to choose from a given set of responses that includes a novel response and at least one familiar response, most nonhuman animals choose randomly, whereas humans tend to choose the novel

A. Ogawa (✉)
RIKEN Brain Science Institute, 2-1 Hirosawa,
Wako, Saitama 351-0198, Japan
e-mail: akitoshi@brain.riken.jp; akitoshi.ogawa@gmail.com

K. Kansaku and L.G. Cohen (eds.), *Systems Neuroscience and Rehabilitation*,
DOI 10.1007/978-4-431-54008-3_9, © Springer 2011

response [1–3]. For example, in an object-naming situation [4–6], when a novel object and a familiar object are presented with a novel label and a familiar label, children tend to assume that the novel label signifies the novel object. This evidently innate tendency leads to rapid lexical learning [4–6]. This response bias is called "exclusion", and it allows us to learn novel relations immediately without repetition [7]. Exclusion appears to be a distinct faculty, not a phenomenon that can be explained by familiarity avoidance or novelty preference (neophilia) [1], both of which are observed in animal studies of exclusion. Exclusion presumes the subjects to choose the familiar label in the presence of familiar object. Exclusion reliably relates the novel label to the novel object, which suggests a cognitive adaptation almost unique to humankind.

Given the relation 'A → B' (if A, then B), three formal variations can be inferred: the inverse, '~A → ~B' (if not A, then not B); the converse, 'B → A'; and the contrapositive, '~B → ~A'. Note that the inverse and converse are, strictly speaking, logically invalid, whereas the contrapositive is valid. Exclusion can encompass all three of these inferred relations, but it appears that a strong bias to infer the converse is a necessary precondition for the ability to practice exclusion. It is well established that when humans learn unidirectional relations (object → label), they immediately convert them into symmetrical, bidirectional relations (object ↔ label). This bias is called "symmetric inference", and it is thought to constitute an important element in the human capacity for naming and labeling. Symmetry can be tested by training a subject to match sample stimulus A to comparison stimulus B, and then testing whether he/she spontaneously matches B as a sample to A as a comparison. A human study suggested that symmetry is deeply related to inference by exclusion [8]. Symmetry is an important criterion for showing exclusion. In two animal studies, one chimpanzee (*Pan troglodytes*) [9, 10] and multiple Californian sea lions (*Zalophus californianus*) [11] displayed exclusion after passing tests for symmetry. However, these examples are exceptional. Other animal studies have failed to show symmetry, even in chimpanzees [12]. These reports suggest that symmetrical inference is an important cognitive process of exclusion. Human subjects, in contrast, readily infer the sample from the familiar comparison. Further, they can easily distinguish a novel sample from the inferred sample. Therefore, human subjects can readily reject the familiar comparison and choose a novel comparison.

A functional magnetic resonance imaging (fMRI) study investigated the neural mechanism associated with exclusion when human subjects performed a matching-to-sample task (Fig. 1). This chapter briefly provides what the fMRI study revealed [13]. The subjects were trained with two unidirectional sample-to-comparison relations: 'S1 → C1' and 'S2 → C2' based on feedback. After training, the subjects were exposed to three tests of stimulus relation involving additional novel stimuli. In the Exclusion test, in which the defined comparison C1 (C2) and the novel comparison N2 (N4) were presented with the novel sample N1 (N3), the subjects were tested whether to reject the defined comparison and choose N2 (N4). The other two tests were control for the Exclusion test. In the S+test, the defined sample S1 (S2) and the defined comparison C1 (C2) were presented with the novel comparison N5 (N6). In the S− test, the novel comparison N7 (N8) was presented with the defined sample

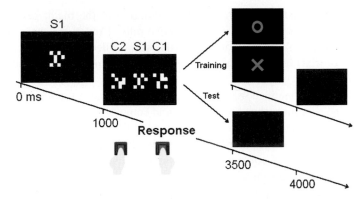

Fig. 1 The time course of a trial. The stimuli appeared near the center of the subject's visual field so that the subject could see them without eye movement. Each trial of the task started with a fixation period, in which the subject fixated on a small white cross that appeared at the center of the display for 1,500 ms. A sample stimulus replaced the fixation cross for 1,000 ms, then two comparison stimuli appeared to the left and right of the sample and persisted for an additional 2,500 ms, after which all stimuli disappeared. The subjects were asked to choose one of the two comparison stimuli by key-press before the stimuli disappeared. In the training session, after the stimuli had disappeared, a feedback – a 'O' for a correct response, or a 'X' for an incorrect response – was presented to the subjects for 500 ms. No feedback was given in the fMRI session. Between trials, the screen was blank for 500 ms in the training session and 1,500–4,500 ms in the test session. (modified from [13])

S1 (S2) and the defined comparison C2 (C1). Note that all three tests tapped the cognitive process of novelty detection, and that the two control tests probed whether the subjects retained the trained relations even when novel comparisons appeared. The activation related to exclusion can be compared with that reported in previous fMRI studies, which suggested that symmetry was performed in the frontoparietal network [14–17].

Experiment

Eighteen right-handed healthy adults with no history of neurological or psychiatric disorders participated in the study, after providing written informed consent. The institutional review board of RIKEN approved the study. The data from three subjects were excluded because of less accuracy. The data from the remaining 15 subjects (seven females, aged 21–36 years) were used for the analysis.

The subjects learned two sample-to-comparison relations in the training session. The stimuli used for each subject were randomly and mutually exclusively selected from the stimulus pool of 15 abstract figures. The time course of a trial is shown in Fig. 1. There were nine rest blocks of 30 s and eight trial blocks of ten trials in training session. There was 10 min break before the test session. In the test session, we used a jittered-event-related design, in which the duration of the blank periods of the inter-trial interval was varied. We conducted two runs of functional scans. Each run contained 80 trials, so a total of 160 trials were collected from each subject. The number of trials for each condition was 20 in each run and the condition order was randomized.

The test session contained four task conditions: Baseline, S+, S−, and Exclusion. In the Baseline condition, the same samples and comparisons as used in the training session were presented. The remaining three conditions were test conditions, and included novel stimuli in addition to learned stimuli. In the S+condition, the same sample stimuli and their corresponding comparison stimuli as those used in the training session were presented, but one of the comparison stimuli was novel and task-irrelevant. With this condition, the subjects were examined whether to retain the stimulus relations even when a novel, irrelevant comparison stimulus was presented. In the S− condition, the same sample stimuli as were used in the training session were presented together with two incorrect comparison stimuli: the comparison stimulus from the other trained relation and a novel comparison stimulus. The subjects were probed whether to have learned to choose the correct comparison by rejecting the irrelevant comparison. In the Exclusion condition, a novel sample stimulus was presented followed by one novel comparison stimulus and one of the trained comparison stimuli. The choice of the novel comparison stimulus was considered "correct." The novel stimuli were counterbalanced across the subjects. Because the cognitive process for novelty detection was common to all test conditions, it was expected to observe brain activity commonly associated with novelty detection, together with activation specifically related to Exclusion.

Results

In the training session, all the subjects achieved the attainment criterion of 85% accuracy (average 92.8%). The response accuracies in the first half (average 86.5%) and the second half (96.5%) of the session were significantly different (paired t test, $t_{14}=3.40$, $P<0.01$). In the test session, one-way repeated-measures analysis of variance (ANOVA) of the reaction time and the response accuracy for the three conditions (Baseline, S+, and Exclusion)[1] showed no significant main effect. Therefore, even though the subjects received no feedback, they consistently and correctly chose the defined comparison stimulus in S+, and consistently and as expected chose a novel comparison stimulus in Exclusion with the same accuracy as in Baseline. The subjects also consistently responded correctly in Baseline. The high accuracy in Exclusion indicated that the relation between the novel sample stimulus and the novel comparison stimulus was immediately inferred and retained during the fMRI scan, consistent with the results of previous studies [1, 4, 5].

---

[1]S− condition was not used in the analysis (Appendix 2).

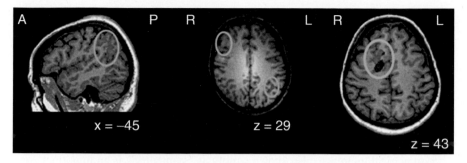

Fig. 2 Imaging result. (*Left, center*) Activation of the 'Exclusion>Baseline' contrast is depicted in the IPL in a sagittal (x=−45) section and in the PFC and IPL in a transaxial (z=29) section. A, anterior; P, posterior; R, right; L, left. (*Right*) The conjunction of the significant activation in the 'Exclusion>Baseline' contrast and the 'S+>Baseline' contrast is depicted on a transaxial (z=43) section

In the analysis of fMRI data in training session, the first four blocks were compared with the last four blocks. The results showed that the activation of the bilateral prefrontal cortex (PFC), right middle temporal gyrus, bilateral middle occipital gyrus, and right lingual gyrus. Exclusion-related brain activation that was analyzed with the contrast 'Exclusion>Baseline' was observed in the right PFC and left inferior parietal lobule [IPL, including the supramarginal gyrus, which extended to the angular gyrus (the temporoparietal junction)]. The 'S+>Baseline' contrast revealed the activation of the right medial frontal cortex (MFC) and the right caudate head The activation in the right MFC partially overlapped with the MFC locus observed in the 'Exclusion>Baseline' contrast (Fig. 2).

Discussion

Significant activation of the right PFC and left IPL was observed in the contrast 'Exclusion>Baseline'. This activation differed most clearly from the activation observed in the contrast 'First Half>Second Half' in the training session, whereas they partly overlapped by 10.7% (by volume) in the right PFC. The overlapping area might be involved in relating the stimuli by learning in the training session and by exclusion in the testing session. These observations suggest that the right PFC and left IPL are not involved in learning, but are instead involved in emergent-relational inference during exclusion. The cognitive process of exclusion consists of several subprocesses: novelty detection, symmetrical inference, and rejection of the defined comparison. The MFC activation observed in both S+ and Exclusion may be associated with novelty detection. Based on that assumption, the observed prefrontal and parietal activation must account for the remaining components of exclusion, namely symmetrical inference and the rejection of the defined comparison.

The activation of the MFC was overlapped between the contrasts 'S+>Baseline' and 'Exclusion>Baseline.' The peak of the BOLD signal of 'Exclusion>Baseline' preceded that of 'S+>Baseline' by 2 s. The first novel stimulus in Exclusion is the sample, whereas the first novel stimulus in S+ is one of the two comparisons, which appears exactly 1,000 ms after the onset of the sample. Because they appeared simultaneously, the subjects may have required additional time to process the novelty or familiarity of the comparisons. Furthermore, the novel stimulus in Exclusion was task-relevant, whereas that in S+ was task-irrelevant. This might have engaged the subjects' attention differently between the two tasks. For these reasons, it is not surprising that the time to recognize novelty was greater in S+ than in Exclusion. It is reasonable to interpret that the MFC is associated with novelty detection.

Symmetrical inference, also known simply as "symmetry", is an important component of the cognitive process of exclusion. When given a conditional relation $(A \rightarrow B)$, humans reflexively infer the converse or symmetric relation $(B \rightarrow A)$, even though this constitutes a logical fallacy. After detecting a novel sample stimulus and a defined comparison stimulus in the Exclusion test, the subjects symmetrically inferred the sample stimulus from the presented defined comparison stimulus. On this basis, they could reject the defined comparison stimulus and choose the novel comparison stimulus. It has been suggested that symmetry plays an important role in word learning by making labels (words) immediately interchangeable with the objects or concepts they represent [4, 5]. Studies of word learning further indicate that symmetry plays an important role when a novel object acquires a label through exclusion [4–6]. Previous fMRI studies have suggested that the prefrontal and parietal cortices are involved in forming abstract categories using symmetry [14–18]. These studies suggest that prefrontal and parietal activation and their functional connection are associated with symmetry, and that symmetry is indeed an important component of exclusion. In line with these fMRI studies, lesion studies suggests that the training of symmetrical inference, a part of exclusion processing, can be useful for rehabilitation of name-face matching [19] and facial-emotional recognition [20].

Evolution has equipped humankind with a suite of cognitive biases that are adaptive and useful cognitive heuristics for everyday decision making. The results suggest that the PFC and the IPL cooperatively support the reasoning by exclusion. The left angular gyrus, part of the IPL, has been shown to be involved in writing and reading [21, 22]. The IPL is also associated with the mental number line [23, 24]. Furthermore, the IPL might be involved in the false belief [25–27]. In short, the IPL appears to be involved in many cognitive functions characteristic to humans. From the view of evolution, macaque monkeys have no homologue of the human IPL [28], suggesting that the evolutionary expansion of the IPL, as well as its connectivity with the PFC, is associated with several vital components of human intelligence.

Appendix 1: Image Acquisition and Analysis

The brain images were collected using a 4 T Varian Unity Inova MRI system. The BOLD signal was measured using a T2*-weighted echo planar imaging sequence (TR = 2,600 ms, TE = 25 ms, FA = 40°). Twenty-five axial slices (thickness = 5.0 mm, gap = 0 mm, FOV = 240 × 240 mm, matrix = 64 × 64) were acquired per volume. A set of high-resolution T1-weighted structural images was obtained by magnetization-prepared 3D FLASH (TR = 110 ms, TE = 6.2 ms, FA = 11°, matrix = 256 × 256 × 180, voxel size = 1 × 1 × 1 mm³).

The functional and structural images were analyzed with Brain Voyager QX. The functional images for each subject were preprocessed, including slice time correction, three-dimensional motion correction, spatial smoothing with a Gaussian filter (FWHM = 6 mm) and high-pass filtering (0.01 Hz). The structural image was transformed into the standard Talairach space. The functional images were transformed into the standard Talairach space by normalizing and resizing them to the transformed structural image. BOLD signals were modeled using a synthetic hemodynamic response function composed of two gamma functions. Random-effects analysis was performed on the functional data to reveal significant activation.

Appendix 2: S– Condition

In S–, a novel comparison replaced the relevant trained comparison, whereas in S+, a novel comparison replaced the trained irrelevant comparison. The S– condition was not used in the analysis because eight subjects did not respond as expected to the S– condition. Four of the subjects chose the defined comparison (C2 was chosen in the presence of S1), whereas the other four subjects responded randomly. To respond accurately, it was necessary to reject the defined comparison and choose the novel one, based on the negative relations of 'if S1, then not C2' and 'if S2, then not C1'. There are two possible explanations for this failure: one is that the training was insufficient, and the other is that the subjects could not reject the defined comparison stimulus. The latter possibility is not plausible, because the subjects rejected the defined comparison stimulus in Exclusion. These results suggest that the subjects did not learn the negative relations sufficiently.

References

1. Aust U, Range F, Steurer M, Huber L (2008) Inferential reasoning by exclusion in pigeons, dogs, and humans. Anim Cogn 11:587–597
2. Beran MJ, Washburn DA (2002) Chimpanzee responding during matching to sample: control by exclusion. J Exp Anal Behav 78:497–508
3. Clement TS, Zentall TR (2003) Choice based on exclusion in pigeons. Psychon Bull Rev 10:959–964
4. Markman EM, Wachtel GF (1988) Children's use of mutual exclusivity to constrain the meanings of words. Cogn Psychol 20:121–157
5. Markman EM, Wasow JL, Hansen MB (2003) Use of the mutual exclusivity assumption by young word learners. Cogn Psychol 47:241–275
6. Piccin TB, Blewitt P (2007) Resource conservation as a basis for the mutual exclusivity effect in children's word learning. First Lang 27:5–28
7. McIlvane WJ, Kledaras JB, Munson LC, King KAJ, Derose JC, Stoddard LT (1987) Controlling relations in conditional discrimination and matching by exclusion. J Exp Anal Behav 48:187–208

8. Stromer R (1989) Symmetry of control by exclusion in humans' arbitrary matching to sample. Psychol Rep 64:915–922

9. Tomonaga M, Matsuzawa T, Fujita K, Yamamoto J (1991) Emergence of symmetry in a visual conditional discrimination by chimpanzees (*Pan troglodytes*). Psychol Rep 68:51–60

10. Tomonaga M (1993) Tests for control by exclusion and negative stimulus relations of arbitrary matching to sample in a symmetry-emergent chimpanzee. J Exp Anal Behav 59:215–229

11. Kastak CR, Schusterman RJ (2002) Sea lions and equivalence: expanding classes by exclusion. J Exp Anal Behav 78:449–465

12. Dugdale N, Lowe CF (2000) Testing for symmetry in the conditional discriminations of language-trained chimpanzees. J Exp Anal Behav 73:5–22

13. Ogawa A, Yamazaki Y, Ueno K, Cheng K, Iriki A (2010) Inferential reasoning by exclusion recruits parietal and prefrontal cortices. Neuroimage 52:1603–1610

14. Dickins DW, Singh KD, Roberts N, Burns P, Downes JJ, Jimmieson P, Bentall RP (2001) An fMRI study of stimulus equivalence. Neuroreport 12:405–411

15. Schlund MW, Hoehn-Saric R, Cataldo MF (2007) New knowledge derived from learned knowledge: functional–anatomic correlates of stimulus equivalence. J Exp Anal Behav 87:287–307

16. Schlund MW, Cataldo MF, Hoehn-Saric R (2008) Neural correlates of derived relational responding on tests of stimulus equivalence. Behav Brain Funct 4:6

17. Ogawa A, Yamazaki Y, Ueno K, Cheng K, Iriki A (2010) Neural correlates of species-typical illogical cognitive bias in human inference. J Cogn Neurosci 22:2120–2130

18. Dickins DW (2005) On aims and methods in the neuroimaging of derived relations. J Exp Anal Behav 84:453–483

19. Cowley BJ, Green G, Braunling-McMorrow D (1992) Using stimulus equivalence procedures to teach name-face matching to adults with brain injuries. J Appl Behav Anal 25:461–475

20. Guercio JM, Podolska-Schroeder H, Rehfeldt RA (2004) Using stimulus equivalence technology to teach emotion recognition to adults with acquired brain injury. Brain Injury 18:593–601

21. Gold M, Adair JC, Jacobs DH, Heilman KM (1995) Right-left confusion in Gerstmann's syndrome – a mode of body-centered spatial orientation. Cortex 31:267–283

22. Horwitz B, Rumsey JM, Donohue BC (1998) Functional connectivity of the angular gyrus in normal reading and dyslexia. Proc Natl Acad Sci USA 95:8939–8944

23. Göbel S, Walsh V, Rushworth M (2001) The mental number line and the human angular gyrus. Neuroimage 14:1278–1289

24. Cattaneo Z, Silvanto J, Pascual-Leone A, Battelli L (2009) The role of the angular gyrus in the modulation of visuospatial attention by the mental number line. Neuroimage 44:563–568

25. Samson D, Apperly IA, Chiavarino C, Humphreys GW (2004) Left temporoparietal junction is necessary for representing someone else's belief. Nat Neurosci 7:499–500

26. Aichhorn M, Perner J, Kronbichler M, Staffen W, Ladurner G (2006) Do visual perspective tasks need theory of mind? Neuroimage 30:1059–1068

27. Perner J, Aichhorn M, Kronbichler M, Staffen W, Ladurner G (2006) Thinking of mental and other representations: the roles of left and right temporo-parietal junction. Soc Neurosci 1:245–258

28. Husain M, Nachev P (2007) Space and the parietal cortex. Trends Cogn Sci 11:30–361 S– condition was not used in the analysis (Appendix 2)

Index

Printed in Japan